Contemporary Chiropractic Philosophy

AN INTRODUCTION

---

*A Reformulation of the Thirty-Three Principles
and the Normal Complete Cycle*

David B. Koch, D.C., D.Ph.C.S.

Professor
Department of Chiropractic Sciences
College of Chiropractic
Life University
Marietta, Georgia

david.koch@life.edu
www.contemporarychiropracticphilosophy.com

Roswell Publishing Company
2300 Holcomb Bridge Road
Suite 103-104
Roswell, GA 30076

ISBN 978-0-9763520-2-0

Manufactured in the United States of America

"Think, damn it, think!"

REGGIE

I dedicate this book to Reggie,
who "turned up the rheostat" of my philosophic mind;

to Dr. Doug Gates,
who suggested to me that perhaps chiropractic's
traditional philosophy could be, and maybe even ought to be,
a completely logically defensible argument;

to the five thousand chiropractic students
and countless chiropractors who, over the last thirty years,
have challenged me to bring clarity to these concepts;

and to Dr. Joe Strauss,
for his encouragement, by suggestion and example, to "get it written."

Thank you.

ACKNOWLEDGEMENTS

When I look back with gratitude over all of those whose help has been invaluable in doing this work, first and foremost, I think of Dr. Guy Riekeman, who, first as one of my teachers at Sherman College, then later during his tenure at Palmer and now at Life University, has given me the unflagging encouragement and support, the resources and, most importantly, the "head-space" necessary for me to give birth to this particular intellectual offspring of mine.

I am deeply indebted, as well, to Dr. Rob Scott, who devoted many hours of his time reading and giving me his input on what I was writing, and who kept assuring me that, yes; it might actually make sense to someone else besides me. I also have to thank him for his critical skepticism and his challenging questions throughout the process of molding thirty years of teaching and lecturing into this, my first volume of philosophic musings.

I wish to give acknowledgement to those many chiropractors, and especially to Drs. Reggie Gold, Thom Gelardi and Fred Barge, who all encouraged me to be bold enough to insist that chiropractic's basic concepts could be updated without necessarily destroying them, in spite of any dogmatic brittleness they may have acquired over the years.

I also want to thank Dr. Brian McAulay for many hours of productive philosophic discussion, and for his work on chiropractic's "Authoritative vs. Dismissive" philosophic impasse which, along with some of Dr. Ian Coulter's writings, has challenged the chiropractic profession to "kick start" the critical philosophic discourse and scholarship so crucial to the survival, growth, and evolution of chiropractic's initial metaphysical insights and vitalistic values.

For the inspiration I take from reading her articles on chiropractic's vitalistic approach to life and health, to make my own writing style a little more humane and approachable, as well as for her help and assistance in formatting, illustrating and preparing my text for publication, and for putting up with me for the last twenty six years, I thank my wonderful wife and life partner, Rebecca.

Isaac Newton said, "If I have seen further it is by standing on the shoulders of giants." When I consider the vantage point on life that chiropractic philosophy has given me, I cannot help but stand in awe of, and therefore acknowledge the profound contributions that the works of Drs. D. D. Palmer, B. J. Palmer, and R. W. Stephenson have made to my life. The view from atop their shoulders appears to me to stretch far beyond anything we have even begun to realize since they strode across the "health care" landscape nearly a century ago. And if my words can help others climb up onto those same tall shoulders and see that same vision of one possible future of human life and health, there will be value enough in them to justify my efforts.

CONTENTS

PART ONE: Chiropractic's "Thirty-Three Principles"

PART TWO: Chiropractic's "Normal Complete Cycle"

PART ONE

Chiropractic's "Thirty-Three Principles"

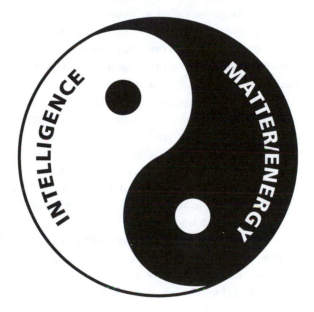

The Material/Immaterial Duality of Existence

CHAPTER 1

Introduction

*All life is an ongoing experiment, and like any good experiment, it exists to explore a basic question, or hypothesis. In fact, every life unfolds to explore the same basic hypothesis, namely, "What unique actions can be expressed through **this particular form of being, this specific confluence of mind and matter?"***

For the last fifty four years, ever since I was two years old, I have been participating in what might be called a "living experiment." As a child, my participation was involuntary. Later, when I became an adult, the experiment itself demanded that I make a conscious choice whether or not, and on what terms, I would be willing to continue participating. I chose to do so. The expected outcome of this "living experiment" involved my own physical, mental, social, even spiritual *state of being* over my entire lifetime.

As with any experiment, there has been a control group, consisting of almost all of my peers. Actually the "control group" could be said to include an entire world full of my fellow human beings. Most of the world's population, either through a lack of awareness or access, or even, occasionally, through a conscious choice, have opted out of my particular experiment. They have been participating, mostly by default, in another, vastly more common "state of being" experiment, which I would characterize as "never having had their spines checked, and adjusted if necessary, by a chiropractor." I use this vocabulary, and make this distinction, because my "living experiment," as all experiments must, involves a *variable,* and that variable is "being under lifetime chiropractic care."

The course of this life-long experiment has been, at its most profound, the experience of living in a state of being that is a consequence of getting my spine checked regularly, and adjusted as needed. Along the way, I also chose to pursue a career as a chiropractor and chiropractic educator. This introduced another layer to my ongoing life experiment, namely the rather odd and most interesting perspective of being both the experimenter and a subject of the same experiment. I remember very clearly an internal experience I had in my student days at Sherman College in the late 1970's, while studying chiropractic philosophy. We were exploring the traditional principles that form the basic metaphor for how chiropractic actually works to help people recover/recreate their own health from within. We heard things like *"Chiropractic gets sick people well, and keeps well people well . . . because . . . The power that made the body heals the body."* We were challenged to consider that if the relative simple act of a well-timed and well-placed chiropractic adjustment could elicit such a profoundly life-changing response from an individual who had already lost his/her health and was sick or dying, how much more potent, constructive and appropriate would it be to adjust vertebral subluxations as soon as they appear, thus allowing individuals and families to live years of greater health and vitality rather than recover from years of mal-adaptation and incoordination. As Reggie (Dr. Reggie Gold) put it, *"I got sick and tired of my patients coming in to my office to get well, and leaving their families at home to get sick."*

Participating in class discussions and reading Stephenson's *Chiropractic Textbook,* I was first introduced to and started to become familiar with chiropractic's "Thirty-Three Principles." As I absorbed the *ideas* that these principles embodied, I realized that they formed the basic substance of a part of my being which was fundamentally different from most of my peers. In fact, it was the very difference that caused me to actually view my life as an experiment and myself as the lab rat. The sensation of consciously examining the very concepts that formed a large part of the heretofore unconscious basis of my worldview actually made my physically dizzy. I remember feeling like my thoughts on chiropractic philosophy were a whirlwind within my own head. Later, as the whirlwind slowed a little, and I started to sort these ideas out, I came to realize that these "principles" also formed a distinct element of the "experiment" itself. Collectively they formed the basic metaphysical *hypothesis* of my chiropractic life!

How can something as simple and undramatic as a chiropractic spinal adjustment...have such a life-altering impact on people's lives?

Simply put, the underlying metaphysical question of my life, as someone who has had ongoing chiropractic care for the location, analysis and adjustment (as needed) of vertebral subluxation throughout life, is, "How can something as simple and undramatic as a chiropractic spinal adjustment, given when and where needed, possess the potential to cause profound and dramatic changes in a person's health, and thereby have such a life-altering impact on people's lives?" How can it be that generation after generation of people, many starting from an attitude of extreme skepticism, have come to view ongoing chiropractic care as one of the very pillars of a healthy state of being?

As a student, I saw this question emerge from the whirlwind of my mind as the central metaphysical issue of the professional vision I was drawn to, namely offering chiropractic care to people as an important and necessary element of a life of optimal health and vitality. In the resonance I felt with this chiropractic per-spective, I recognized that, like most chiropractic students, I was simply seeing chiropractic through the prism of my own experience of lifelong chiropractic care. But considering that lifelong chiropractic care for everyone would *include* chiropractic care for anyone for whom a timely chiropractic adjustment might have value as an episodic intervention, this perspective seemed then, and still seems today, like the most potentially beneficial, economical and effective approach to what chiropractic as a profession *could be.*

As a chiropractic educator, I soon discovered that the very question that had emerged as the central issue in my mind when I was a student was also the most pressing question I was being asked to explore with *my* students, except that, in their case, as it was with me as a practicing chiropractor, the significance of the question was not "Why can the adjustment have such an impact on my own life?" Rather, it was "Why does such a little thing that *I can do for another person* have the potential to elicit such a powerful, often unpredictable, sometimes overwhelming response from them?" After all, a single chiropractic adjustment isn't really that involved an interaction. It doesn't take a lot of time, or require a lot of energy to accomplish. It doesn't even require that the chiropractor neces-sarily understands how the person he/she is adjusting is going to react to the adjustment, or that the person receiving the adjustment even understands what is happening.[1] How can these things occur? What power or potential does the adjustment allow the person receiving it to tap into *within him/herself?*

With students, the question of the source of the potential power of the spinal adjustment, upon which we are asking them to build their professional career, becomes a question of *trust,* as well as one of intellectual curiosity. To the "fledgling chiropractor," chiropractic's basic principles seem to suggest that, con-trary to the prevailing "health care" paradigm in which patients are asked to trust the doctor, or the surgeon, or the procedure, or the drug, or even the phar-maceutical company itself, in fact, to trust virtually anyone but themselves for their "cure," the chiropractor has to actually *trust the patient,* and more specifi-cally the patient's own body, for the solution to the patient's problem. This means that the source of the potential power of the spinal adjustment lies not with the adjustic thrust that the chiropractor delivers, but with the ability of the person receiving the adjustic thrust both to make the actual adjustment itself and to create health within his/her own body, where before there was incoordi-nation, dysfunction and mal-adaptation. In other words, the chiropractor has to *give up* his/her power over the other person's life in order to facilitate and max-imize *the expression of that person's own natural ability to control, regulate, create,*

---

[1] Consider that chiropractic adjustments often elicit tremendous, life changing, healing and/or health enhancing responses from uncomprehending babies and even animals.

adapt, evolve and re-create (heal/repair) him/herself. Actually, chiropractic has trusted, and worked with, this natural ability, referred to as the body's *innate intelligence,* since its inception.

This can be a difficult attitudinal transition for anyone, and especially for students, to make. As a society, we are so completely immersed in the attitude that diseases and symptoms are enemies to be fought, that we often find ourselves fighting not only against the microbial environment in which we live and which lives within us, but also against our own bodies' best efforts to function and adapt effectively and efficiently in relationship to the environment. This is particularly true when the body's adaptive efforts and strategies involve the unusual and uncomfortable states of being we think of as symptoms. Yet we really know that we cannot ultimately

> **Chiropractic has trusted, and worked with, this natural ability, referred to as the body's *innate intelligence,* since its inception.**

win an all-out war with our microbial neighbors; even today we are seeing them (the microbes) get stronger as we get weaker. The noted French M.D./microbiologist Rene Dubois perhaps said it best when he pointed out that all a microbial infection really demonstrates is that there has been a "failure of negotiations between man and the microbial world."[2] And we only compound the problem when we fight against, suppress and deny our own bodies' adaptive responses.

Then, right into the middle of this warfare mentality, along comes chiropractic's basic principles, suggesting that maybe people don't really need to find and hire better disease fighters. Maybe they need to *become better self-healers.* Could chiropractic really be saying that people, struggling to adapt to the challenges of living, actually need to put more *trust* in the inborn wisdom *(innate intelligence)* of life itself, and in the body's ability to heal itself in its own way and at its own pace, than in the entire resources of the medical profession, acting as hired guns ready to do battle with their diseases? Can the student accept that putting *complete unqualified trust* in the patient's own *innate intelligence* to do the real work at hand, to meet the adaptive challenge, to fight the immunological fight, to reconstruct the damaged and broken body, is a *reasonable attitude* to entertain? Can the practicing chiropractor *responsibly claim* that, as a consequence of a simple but thorough spinal examination for vertebral subluxation, and the delivery of spinal adjustments when and where they are needed, a newborn may thrive instead of just survive, an athlete may run faster, jump higher, maybe even win the gold metal instead of the silver, a person fighting for his/her life with a malignant tumor growing within may be able to fight just a little harder, and astound the medical profession with yet another unexpected spontaneous

[2] R. Dubois' *Man Adapting*

remission? Can we *better* help meet humanity's needs by being quiet, humble *change agents* for health, rather than *warrior champions* on the battlefield of disease? Sometimes this can truly be a difficult transition to make. As D. D. Palmer[3] put it in 1910, *"Those who expect to put in a life-time combating disease, fighting the entrance of disease, as tho it was an enemy with hostile intent, should not learn Chiropractic. It is very difficult to change a medical warrior into a peaceful Chiropractor."*[4] As I said, there was a whirlwind in my head.

> **"Those who expect to put in a life-time combating disease, fighting the entrance of disease, as tho it was an enemy with hostile intent, should not learn Chiropractic. It is very difficult to change a medical warrior into a peaceful Chiropractor."**
>
> **D. D. PALMER (1910)**

For me, the answers to these questions and many others that I had about the very life I was living lay in my exploration and clear understanding of what these basic chiropractic principles meant and implied. For me, the *justification* of the trust I placed in my own body's natural wisdom and capacity for self-creation, self-maintenance, self-repair and self-evolution, and that I was proposing others, both my students and my patients, should place in themselves and their own capacities, was embodied in these principles that I read in Stephenson's *Chiropractic Textbook,* and lectured on, and thought about, and examined for their meaningfulness. For me, the vision that formed in my mind, and that I hold to this day, of a world in which, someday, probably not within my own lifetime, but perhaps within the foreseeable future of the human species, every human being might have the opportunity to choose to live the "life experiment" that I was living, emerged from the simple assumption and conclusions that constituted what I had learned and have taught as chiropractic philosophy.

Now it has become my responsibility to try to help pass on these very fertile and formative ideas that I have found to be so rich in meaning, and so *trustworthy,* to others. I do not propose that I have understood them where others have not, or that my reasoned reformulation of them or my explanations of their many meanings are better or more important than those of others who have sought to further illuminate them and spread the message they hold. But I do propose to help deepen their impact by improving their structure and form, through my own best effort at a rigorous critical analysis of their conceptual content and a willingness to update the very words, ordering and logical consistency that gives these principles their meaning, and therefore their meaningfulness and usefulness, to those of us who will ultimately succeed, or fail, in our "life experiment" involving that "state of being" attainable only through a life-

---

[3] Daniel David Palmer, Discoverer of Chiropractic, 1845-1913
[4] D. D. Palmer's *The Chiropractor's Adjuster,* p. 117

long commitment to *living chiropractic lives* ourselves and *bringing chiropractic care* to others.

CHAPTER 2

Stephenson's Thirty-Three Principles

Chiropractic, like other sciences, has many principles. Some of the principles are basic, upon which others are founded or derived as going from the general to the specific; some are down to a part of the whole thing. These specific principles are of course derived principles. They are not limited to any given number.

R. W. STEPHENSON (1927)

Considering the role its philosophy plays in a profession and the various contributions chiropractic philosophy has made and should continue to make to our profession, it is important to consider the nature of the philosophical model on which chiropractic operates. It can be argued that the historic development of what we might call a specific "chiropractic philosophy" centered on the "List of Thirty-Three Principles, numbered and named"[5] in Stephenson's *Chiropractic Textbook*. Therefore, to further the discussion and critical evaluation of chiropractic philosophy, we must first look at and attempt to understand the intrinsic nature, meaning and potential limitations of Stephenson's seminal work. It will be helpful for the reader to spend some time reviewing the Thirty-Three Principles in the introduction,[6] as well as in the Senior Text[7] of Stephenson's *Chiropractic Textbook,* to receive maximum benefit from the following discussion.

One of the first things we discover, as we review our source, is that R. W. Stephenson, in his own conception of how the student might use his "list of Thirty-Three Principles, numbered and named," seemed to think of them primarily as a list of discussion topics. He appears to have been either unaware of their possible interpretation as a sequential logical argument, i.e. a *syllogism,* or perhaps he felt he was neither qualified nor prepared to defend them as such. In fact, a brief look at the history of the relationship between the chiropractic profession and the Thirty-Three Principles over the last eighty years points to an interpretation of these principles not as the discrete steps of a continuous logical structure, but more typically as a collection of separate and distinct, but closely related laws or rules describing the behavior of an "intelligent" universe on both macroscopic and local scales. In this interpretation, Stephenson's Principles would

---

[5] Stephenson's *Chiropractic Textbook,* p. xxxi
[6] Stephenson's *Chiropractic Textbook,* p. xiii-xxxiii
[7] Stephenson's *Chiropractic Textbook,* p. 236-273, 295-335

be similar to other collections of principles like the Ten Commandments or the Bill of Rights. This concept can be illustrated by a scenario where a chiropractor is saying to a patient, "Well, Ms. Jones, according to Principle 6 – The Principle of Time – your baby's fever may take a while to ease off, but please don't worry too much. Remember, Principle 27 – The Normality of Innate Intelligence – teaches us that, as long as we have corrected your baby's subluxations and Innate Intelligence is in control of the body's responses, that fever is just a normal adaptive response."

This interpretation seems to be in keeping with Stephenson's definition of "principles" in the introductory articles leading up to the Principles themselves. In Article 22 – Principle[8] he offers several definitions of the term, including "A fundamental truth; a comprehensive law or doctrine from which others are derived, or on which others are founded; a general truth; an elementary proposition; a maxim; an axiom; a postulate." He then goes on to say, **"The principles of a science are its governing laws.** These may be **the fundamental truths upon which it is founded, or the governing rules of conduct or operation."** In the following article, titled "The Principles of Chiropractic," he describes his principles this way:

"Art. 23. The Principles of Chiropractic

Chiropractic like other sciences, has many principles. As in other sciences some of these principles are different from the rest; some being more fundamental than others. This fact can be seen by examining the foregoing definitions of principles. Some of the principles are basic, upon which others are founded or derived as going from the general to the specific; some are down to a part of the whole thing. These specific principles are of course derived principles. They are not limited to any given number. **A fundamental principle of Chiropractic is a statement of the quality or actions of intelligence in matter which will include any and all circumstances that may arise in study.**

Immediately following are a number of principles which have been chosen for discussion in this book. These are stated and numbered for convenience so that their application to things under discussion can be seen. They are arranged in an order which goes from the general to the specific. They are referred to by number in the text, of which each Article is supported by one or more principles, thereby giving the entire work unity and agreement."[9]

---

[8] Stephenson's *Chiropractic Textbook*, p. *xxix*
[9] Stephenson's *Chiropractic Textbook*, p. *xxx*

If this is, in fact, the scope and intent of Stephenson's Thirty-Three Principles, and the extent of their intrinsic value, then they do *not* constitute the foundation of *the* philosophy of chiropractic or even *a* philosophy of chiropractic. More correctly, we could say that they would in fact be, and therefore deserve to be thought of as, what they have become by reputation, namely a kind of chiropractic creed, or catechism, to be revered and preserved as the unalterable, sacred dogma of the profession. Unfortunately, this would also tend to elevate them above intellectual criticism and arrest their potential development as a useful philosophic model that can evolve along with our knowledge and understanding of the world.

However, a closer reading of this article suggests that Stephenson was hinting at the interpretation of these principles as a true syllogism, even if he didn't realize it! He notes that some of the principles are "basic, upon which others are founded or derived" and that they are "arranged in an order that goes from the general to the specific." He ends with the claim that each Article in the ensuing text "is supported by one or more principles, thereby giving the entire work unity and agreement." All of these descriptions certainly suggest the idea that Stephenson's "Principles of Chiropractic" form some sort of unified rational argument for an internally consistent and, one might add, clearly metaphysical model of reality that would underlie and support chiropractic's inside-out approach to questions of human function and mal-function. This suggestion of a philosophically rigorous model is perhaps most seductively dangled before the profession by Stephenson in the act of naming his first principle the Major Premise of chiropractic. A *major premise* is typically the first assumption of a well-constructed logical syllogism, and forms the foundational basis of all deductions and conclusions that follow. On this basis, it would seem that Stephenson's Principles may well form a viable starting point for just such a rigorous logical exercise.

> A "major premise" is the first assumption of a well-constructed logical syllogism, and forms the foundational basis of all deductions and conclusions that follow.

In examining this possibility, let us begin with an evaluation of Stephenson's Thirty-Three Principles from the point of view of how well they work as a logical metaphysical model of reality. This examination may suggest many possible questions, including:

• Are the Thirty-Three Principles fundamentally deductive?

• Do they follow each other in a logically sensible order?

• Which of them are assumptions, and which are derived conclusions?

• Are the assumptions well-stated, complete, explicit and defensible?

- Are they true? (In other words, do we wish to make these assumptions and then reason from them *as if* they were true?)

- Are the conclusions we draw from them both logically and sensibly meaningful?

- What further assumptions do these conclusions suggest?

- Are any additional assumptions we find in the syllogism congruent with the initial assumptions upon which the argument is being built?

- Do the words and terms Stephenson used still mean the same things they meant in 1927?

- Are there other words and terms we could use to capture Stephenson's meaning more clearly in the context of today's scientific and philosophic thought about the universe?

- Are there any issues or elements of the model that need further elucidation?

- Is the model complete, or are there other assumptions we need to consider, or other conclusions we need to draw to fill out the model?

- If considered as elements of a logical structure, do these principles, when considered in their entirety, form the outline of a model of the basic nature of reality that we can understand.

- Does this model have any applicability to issues of human life, function and health that we, as chiropractors, care about?

All of this may sound like a tall order of business, but it remains the inescapable responsibility of chiropractic's philosophers to consider these questions if we are going to claim that chiropractic's traditional philosophy brings a valuable and defining perspective to the profession. To start to answer these questions, let us begin with Stephenson's original words:

ART. 24. A LIST OF THIRTY-THREE PRINCIPLES, numbered and named.[10]

No. 1. The Major Premise.
> A Universal Intelligence is in all matter and continually gives to it all its properties and actions, thus maintaining it in existence.

No. 2. The Chiropractic Meaning of Life.
> The expression of this intelligence through matter is the Chiropractic meaning of life.

No. 3. The Union of Intelligence and Matter.
> Life is necessarily the union of intelligence and matter.

---

[10] Stephenson's *Chiropractic Textbook*, p. *xxxi-xxxiii*

No. 4. The Triune of Life.
Life is a triunity having three necessary united factors, namely, Intelligence, Force and Matter.

No. 5. The Perfection of the Triune.
In order to have 100% Life, there must be 100% Intelligence, 100% Force, 100% Matter.

No. 6. The Principle of Time.
There is no process that does not require time.

No. 7. The Amount of Intelligence in Matter.
The amount of intelligence for any given amount of matter is 100%, and is always proportional to its requirements.

No. 8. The Function of Intelligence.
The function of intelligence is to create force.

No. 9. The Amount of Force Created by Intelligence.
The amount of force created by intelligence is always 100%.

No. 10. The Function of Force.
The function of force is to unite intelligence and matter.

No. 11. The Character of Universal Forces.
The forces of Universal Intelligence are manifested by physical laws; are unswerving and unadapted, and have no solitude for the structures in which they work.

No. 12. Interference with Transmission of Universal Forces.
There can be interference with transmission of universal forces.

No. 13. The Function of Matter.
The function of matter is to express force.

No. 14. Universal Life.
Force is manifested by motion in matter; all matter has motion, therefore there is universal life in all matter.

No. 15. No Motion without the Effort of Force.
Matter can have no motion without the application of force by intelligence.

No. 16. Intelligence in both Organic and Inorganic Matter.
Universal Intelligence gives force to both organic and inorganic matter.

No. 17. Cause and Effect.
Every effect has a cause and every cause has effects.

No. 18. Evidence of Life.
The signs of life are evidence of the intelligence of life.

No. 19. Organic Matter.
The material of the body of a "living thing" is organized matter.

No. 20. Innate Intelligence.
A "living thing" has an inborn intelligence within its body, called Innate Intelligence.

No. 21. The Mission of Innate Intelligence.
The mission of Innate Intelligence is to maintain the material of the body of a "living thing" in active organization.

No. 22. The Amount of Innate Intelligence.
There is 100% of Innate Intelligence in every "living thing," the requisite amount, proportional to its organization.

No. 23. The Function of Innate Intelligence.
The function of Innate Intelligence is to adapt universal forces and matter for use in the body, so that all parts of the body will have co-ordinated action for mutual benefit.

No. 24. The Limits of Adaptation.
Innate Intelligence adapts forces and matter for the body as long as it can do so without breaking a universal law, or Innate Intelligence is limited by the limitations of matter.

No. 25. The Character of Innate Forces.
The forces of Innate Intelligence never injure or destroy the structures in which they work.

No. 26. Comparison of Universal and Innate Forces.
In order to carry on the universal cycle of life, Universal forces are destructive, and Innate forces constructive, as regards structural matter.

No. 27. The Normality of Innate Intelligence.
Innate Intelligence is always normal and its function is always normal.

No. 28. The Conductors of Innate Forces.
The forces of Innate Intelligence operate through or over the nervous system in animal bodies.

No. 29. Interference with Transmission of Innate Forces.
There can be interference with the transmission of Innate forces.

No. 30. The Causes of Dis-ease.
Interference with the transmission of Innate forces causes incoordination of dis-ease.

No. 31. Subluxations.
Interference with transmission in the body is always directly or indirectly due to subluxations in the spinal column.

No. 32. The Principle of Coordination.
Coordination is the principle of harmonious action of all the parts of an organism, in fulfilling their offices and purposes.

No. 33. The Law of Demand and Supply.
The Law of Demand and Supply is existent in the body in its ideal state; wherein the "clearing house" is the brain, Innate the virtuous "banker," brain cells "clerks," and nerve cells "messengers."

CHAPTER 3

The "Universal Principles"

Today there is a wide measure of agreement, which on the physical side approaches unanimity, that the stream of knowledge is heading toward a non-mechanical realty; the universe begins to look more like a great thought than a great machine.

SIR JAMES JEANS (1932)

A t first glance, this list of sentences with fancy titles may look like just that – a list. But if one takes the time to read through them several times, and it is highly recommend that you do so, some aspects of their deeper order and intrinsic internal structure start to emerge. We notice that they are somewhat linear, starting as they do with "Universal Intelligence" creating universal forces throughout the entire universe, and working all the way down to conclusions concerning the spinal column, the nervous system and subluxations, which are features of specific forms of life, namely us, on a specific planet, namely our own.

We can see clearly that they are related to each other in conceptual groupings. For example, the first seventeen principles, with the exception of Principles 2 through 5, all seem to address the issue of the "intelligence in all matter," and how the forces this universal intelligence creates are manifested as the physical laws affecting all the matter of the universe. Within this conceptual grouping, Principles 2 through 5 seem to be misplaced, since they address the question of what constitutes "life," and we have every reason to believe, considering the principles that follow the first fifteen, that the "life" these subsequent principles address in great detail is organic, biological life.

In fact, this odd juxtaposition of principles that appear to describe the concept of "life" in the midst of a set of principles that seem to apply to the universe as a whole, may cause us to question the placement of Principle 14 (Universal Life – *Force is manifested by motion in matter; all matter has motion, therefore there is **universal life(?)** in all matter.*) as well. Its use of the term "universal life" seems to imply that Stephenson wants to use the term "life" in two different ways, referring to both the "expression of intelligence" in the simple organization inherent in the basic existence of all matter, and the "expression of intelligence" in the highly complex state of dynamic organizational flux, characterized by the interactive coordination of internal functions and continuous adaptations to changing external conditions, which we traditionally think of as "life." This use of the term "life" to signify the organizational expression of intelligence on a universal scale, as well as within the subset of organization represented by the concept of biological life, becomes the first of several major obstacles to seeing and understanding the syllogistic logic and flow implied within the Thirty-Three Principles. Thus, the need to clarify the term "life" may be considered the first necessary step in a philosophic criticism of Stephenson's Principles.

The simplest way to eliminate this double use of the term "life," and begin to clarify Stephenson's Principles, is to exchange it for another term in the concept of "universal life," and reserve the term "life" exclusively for the biological phenomena it traditionally denotes. The other term we should use to express the concept of "universal life" is clearly the term "organization" itself. If the universe's "universal intelligence" is assumed to be the cause of the properties and actions of *all matter,* and not just the properties and actions of living organisms, then its expression in all matter can be said to be represented by the state of organization of any and all forms of matter. This is obvious from the fact that the properties and actions of matter in any of its forms, whether living or not, whether solid, liquid, gas or plasma, at any level of consideration from the subatomic to the galactic, are the consequence of the specific organizational state of the matter we are considering. Physically, even life itself exists as a specific organizational state (admittedly highly complex and dynamic) of specific material elements. Thus, if we wish to refer to the expression of "universal intelligence" in any and all matter, or in the universe as a whole, we are referring to the specific and particular state of *organization* of any particular bit of matter, or of the universe as a whole.

> **Physically, even life itself exists as a specific organizational state (admittedly highly complex and dynamic) of specific material elements.**

Furthermore, if we consider replacing the term "life" with the term "organization" in Principle 14, we must also evaluate the universal, as opposed to the specifically biological, applicability of Principle 4 (The Triune of Life – *Life is a tri-unity having three necessary united factors, namely, Intelligence, Force and Matter.*) Again, if we look at the meaning of the principle, especially in terms of the implications of Principle 14 (above), we quickly conclude that this principle also uses the term "life" in the more general meaning of "universal life." Thus it is also reasonable to consider exchanging the term "organization" for the term "life" in this principle, as well. If we do so *(Organization is a triunity having three necessary united factors, namely, Intelligence, Force and Matter.)*, Principle 4 clearly becomes a universal, not just a biological, principle, and as such should remain where Stephenson originally placed it, rather than being moved down the list with Principles 2, 3 and 5.

To reiterate: we will transpose Principles 2, 3 and 5 further down the list, and substitute the term "organization" for the term "life" in Principles 4 and 14, to indicate the expression of "universal intelligence" in any and all states of material existence. After doing so, we will reserve the term "life" specifically to denote those complex, organic, interactive, adaptive states of organization we intuitively recognize and traditionally designate as "organic" or "biological" life. These changes create a subset of Stephenson's list of principles (Principles 1, 4, and 6–17) that outlines a model of how the entire universe becomes and remains organized, based on the assumption that its organization is the consequence of the continuous and ongoing action of an organizing intelligence. This subset of principles, which we have isolated from the entire list specifically on the basis of their universal applicability, can be categorized as the **universal principles** of Stephenson's list. With this categorization, we create a "syllogism within the syllogism," which can be considered as a separate logical argument unto itself, available for us to evaluate, advance and perfect as best we can.

> With this categorization, we create a "syllogism within the syllogism," which can be considered as a separate logical argument unto itself.

At this point, let's consolidate and reformat this "universal syllogism" that has emerged by the identification and rearrangement of those of Stephenson's principles which are specifically universal in scope. The slight change in the wording of Principles 4 and 14 (the use of the term *organization* in place of the term *life)*, necessary to justify their inclusion in these universal principles, has been indicated with *italics*.

No. 1. The Major Premise.
A Universal Intelligence is in all matter and continually gives to it all its properties and actions, thus maintaining it in existence.

No. 4. The Triune of *Organization.*
Organization is a triunity having three necessary united factors, namely, Intelligence, Force and Matter.

No. 6. The Principle of Time.
There is no process that does not require time.

No. 7. The Amount of Intelligence in Matter.
The amount of intelligence for any given amount of matter is 100%, and is always proportional to its requirements.

No. 8. The Function of Intelligence.

The function of intelligence is to create force.

No. 9. The Amount of Force Created by Intelligence.

The amount of force created by intelligence is always 100%.

No. 10. The Function of Force.

The function of force is to unite intelligence and matter.

No. 11. The Character of Universal Forces.

The forces of Universal Intelligence are manifested by physical laws; are unswerving and unadapted, and have no solitude for the structures in which they work.

No. 12. Interference with Transmission of Universal Forces.

There can be interference with transmission of universal forces.

No. 13. The Function of Matter.

The function of matter is to express force.

No. 14. Universal *Organization*.

Force is manifested by motion in matter; all matter has motion, therefore there is universal *organization* in all matter.

No. 15. No Motion without the Effort of Force.

Matter can have no motion without the application of force by intelligence.

No. 16. Intelligence in both Organic and Inorganic Matter.

Universal Intelligence gives force to both organic and inorganic matter.

No. 17. Cause and Effect.

Every effect has a cause and every cause has effects.

CHAPTER 4

Rearranging the Universal Principles

Putting the cart before the horse frustrates neither the cart nor the horse, but it does tend to frustrate the driver. As we drive our own thinking through logical argumentation, let's get our carts and our horses in the right order, so they can all pull together.

Having assembled those principles which are universal in scope into a separate list, our next step is to analyze them in terms of their integrity as a logical argument. This will constitute two separate and distinct processes. The first will be to examine the specific arrangement of the universal principles in terms of their deductive sequence. In any deductive argument, we are reasoning from premises (assumptions) to conclusions. If these principles do, in fact, constitute any sort of valid syllogism, its validity will only emerge if we identify our initial assumptions, place them first in the syllogism, and order the subsequent principles in deductive sequence. As we begin this process, it will quickly become necessary to keep track of where a principle is located in Stephenson's original ordering and where it is going in our final arrangement. To facilitate clarity during this process, we will refer to principles by their original numbering in Stephenson's *Chiropractic Textbook* with the label "SP_n" throughout the rest of the text, and refer to principles as they are rearranged by the number of their final location.

> **If these principles do, in fact, constitute any sort of valid syllogism, its validity will only emerge if we identify our initial assumptions, place them first in the syllogism, and order the subsequent principles in deductive sequence.**

In considering which of the universal principles are primary *(a priori)* assumptions and which are derived conclusions, three of these principles emerge, identified clearly by their content, although not by their position, as initial presuppositions. These are SP_1, SP_6 and SP_{17}! SP_1 (The Major Premise – *A Universal Intelligence is in all matter and continually gives to it all its properties and actions, thus maintaining it in existence.*) is properly identified by Stephenson as, and will remain, the initial assumption of the entire syllogism. However, it is clearly not the *only* assumption upon which the syllogism is built. SP_6 (The Principle of Time – *There is no process which does not require time.*) is also such a basic assumption about the essential nature of reality that it needs to be placed at the beginning of the syllogism. When we acknowledge the primacy of time, we also immediately realize that the assumption of a temporally unfolding universe leads directly to the identification of a third primary assumption in our "list" of universal principles, namely SP_{17} (Cause and Effect – *Every effect has a cause and every cause has effects.*)

We have identified both of these principles (SP_6 and SP_{17}) as primary assumptions, needing to be placed at the front of the syllogism in order to better define the presuppositions from which the other principles flow, just by looking down our list of principles from first to last, and our temptation might be to place them in the same order at the front of the list (SP_1, SP_6, SP_{17}). However, if we look at the relationship between the concepts of temporal progression and "cause and effect" relationships, one could argue that the passage of time can be *defined* by the "cause and effect" nature of physical processes, rather than the "cause and effect" nature of physical processes being defined by the passage of time. Consequently, we will bring these two principles to the front of the syllogism, and transpose them at the same time, making the assumption of "cause and effect" our second principle, and the implied temporal nature of all "cause and effect" processes our third. Thus, our first three principles become Principle 1 – The Major Premise (SP_1), Principle 2 – Cause and Effect (SP_{17}), and Principle 3 – The Principle of Time (SP_6). By arranging SP_{17} and SP_6 to immediately follow Principle 1, this order contributes to, rather than obscures, the logical progression of the emerging "universal syllogism" and argument.

> **The passage of time can be *defined by* the "cause and effect" nature of physical processes.**

The Concept of Force:

The process of rearrangement continues with the solution to the problem inherent in SP_4 (The Triune of Organization – *Organization is a triunity having three necessary united factors, namely, Intelligence, Force and Matter.*), which we left in its original position as a universal principle, after replacing the term "life" with "organization" (see above). In this position in the syllogism, it appears to be simply a fourth assumption, which introduces the very significant term "force" for the first time. However, as an assumption it is very weak, since it neither implies the derivation nor gives a hint as to the meaning of the very term it introduces, namely *force*. Nor does it illuminate what it is about the relationship between intelligence and matter that necessarily involves the idea of force, as the principle presupposes.

On the other hand, if we examine the rest of the list, we discover that there are two later principles that actually do address the derivation and meaning of the term "force" and its relationship to "intelligence" and "matter." They are SP_{14} (Universal Organization – *Force is manifested by motion in matter; all matter has motion, therefore there is universal organization in all matter.),* and SP_{15} (No Motion without the Effort of Force – *Matter can have no motion without the application of force by intelligence.)* These two principles, as the necessary logical antecedents to SP_4, should therefore be brought forward to precede it in the syllogism.

As was the case with SP_6 (Time) and SP_{17} (Cause and Effect) (see above), we again find that these principles (SP_{14} and SP_{15}) are both out of position *and* out of order. If we bring them forward *and* reverse their order, SP_{15} (No Motion without the Effort of Force) becomes Principle 4, and SP_{14} (Universal Organization) becomes Principle 5. This pushes SP_4 (The Triune of Organization) down to Principle 6, where it becomes the deductive conclusion of the preceding principles, rather than an assumption in its own right. Of course, in doing so we must also consider whether SP_{15} (now our Principle 4) is a fourth assumption or a valid conclusion from the first three assumptions, a question we will explore later on, after we finish arranging the syllogism into a logically defensible deductive sequence, and begin to examine its validity and meaning.

The Triune of Organization:

Next, we find a series of principles that follow each other in what appears to be a strong linear fashion, and consequently need little, if any, refinement of their logical flow. These are SP_7 (The Amount of Intelligence in Matter), SP_8 (The Function of Intelligence), SP_9 (The Amount of Force Created by Intelligence), SP_{10} (The Function of Force), SP_{11} (The Character of Universal Forces), SP_{12} (Interference with Transmission of Universal Forces) and SP_{13} (The Function of Matter). All of these principles serve to illuminate SP_4 (The Triune of Organization), now the sixth principle in our syllogism. The backbone of this argument consists of three principles, SP_8 (The Function of Intelligence), SP_{10} (The Function of Force) and SP_{13} (The Function of Matter). These three key principles are each main definitional statements that flesh out the "triune of organization" *(Organization is a triunity having three necessary united factors, namely, Intelligence, Force and Matter.)* Together, they form the main model of material/immaterial interaction that substantiates the whole syllogism, and serves as the primary doctrine of traditional chiropractic philosophy, known as The Triune of Life.

Logically, it would appear that our argument might be best served if we placed the three main principles in their natural and traditional order, and then placed each of the other principles on the list under the main principle to which it is related. Thus SP_7 (The Amount of Intelligence in Matter) would be placed *under* SP_8 (The Function of Intelligence), making SP_8 Principle 7 and SP_7 Principle 8 in our new order. Similarly, SP_9 (The Amount of Force Created by Intelligence) would go *under* SP_{10} (The Function of Force), along with SP_{11} (The Character of Universal Forces) and SP_{12} (Interference with the Transmission of Universal Forces), which are already in their natural deductive positions. This results in SP_{10} becoming Principle 9, followed by SP_9, SP_{11}, and SP_{12} as Principles 10, 11 and 12. Stephenson's thirteenth principle (The Function of Matter) simply remains in its original position as Principle 13.

Finally, since we moved SP_{14} and SP_{15} forward and transposed them to become Principle 4 and Principle 5 in our new arrangement (see above), SP_{16} (Intelligence in both Organic and Inorganic Matter), the last of our universal principles, stays in its original position, renumbered as Principle 14. This principle now constitutes the final step of our "universal syllogism" and forms an ideal logical bridge *(Universal Intelligence gives force to both **organic** and inorganic matter)* to the next body of principles, which will deal with the question of "life" first alluded to in this principle with its reference to "organic" matter.

The Universal Principles Rearranged:

These suggested rearrangements produce the following list, which begins to look like an orderly argument for the nature of the relationship between intelligence, force and matter. For the purpose of further exploring the nature and meaning of these principles, we will consider them in the order developed above, which will serve two purposes. First, it will allow us to better appreciate that this is *not* just a "list of Principles, named and numbered," as Stephenson originally labeled them. It is a rich and elegant metaphysical model of the basic working mechanism of a presumed intelligent universe, truly a "universal syllogism" as referred to above. Secondly, the ordering of these principles will better reveal their internal connections, relationships and progression, which will ultimately serve to allow us to better understand their meaning and apply that meaning to our own lives and our chiropractic endeavors.

> This is not just a "list of Principles, named and numbered," as Stephenson originally labeled them. It is a rich and elegant metaphysical model of the basic working mechanism of a presumed "intelligent universe."

As we have rearranged those of Stephenson's principles which are universal in scope, it has been necessary to renumber them in the order that appears most meaningful and logically defensible. In order to maintain continuity with Stephenson's work, as the first definitive codification of this chiropractic syllogism, the original identity of each principle's position in Stephenson's original list will be preserved (SP_1, SP_2, etc.) but to avoid future confusion, they will be referred to by their position on this revised list (Principle n) for the rest of this discussion. Any and all changes in wording will continue to be indicated with *italics*.

STEPHENSON'S "UNIVERSAL PRINCIPLES" IN LOGICAL ORDER

No. 1. The Major Premise. (SP_1)
A Universal Intelligence is in all matter and continually gives to it all its properties and actions, thus maintaining it in existence.

No. 2. Cause and Effect. (SP_{17})
Every effect has a cause and every cause has effects.

No. 3. The Principle of Time. (SP_6)
There is no process that does not require time.

No. 4. No Motion without the Effort of Force. (SP_{15})
Matter can have no motion without the application of force by intelligence.

No. 5. Universal *Organization*. (SP_{14})
Force is manifested by motion in matter; all matter has motion, therefore there is universal *organization* in all matter.

No. 6. The Triune of *Organization*. (SP_4)
Organization is a triunity having three necessary united factors, namely, Intelligence, Force and Matter.

No. 7. The Function of Intelligence. (SP_8)
The function of intelligence is to create force.

No. 8. The Amount of Intelligence in Matter. (SP_7)
The amount of intelligence for any given amount of matter is 100%, and is always proportional to its requirements.

No. 9. The Function of Force. (SP_{10})
The function of force is to unite intelligence and matter.

No. 10. The Amount of Force Created by Intelligence. (SP_9)
The amount of force created by intelligence is always 100%.

No. 11. The Character of Universal Forces. (SP_{11})
The forces of Universal Intelligence are manifested by physical laws; are unswerving and unadapted, and have no solitude for the structures in which they work.

No. 12. Interference with Transmission of Universal Forces. (SP_{12})
There can be interference with transmission of universal forces.

No. 13. The Function of Matter. (SP_{13})
The function of matter is to express force.

No. 14. Intelligence in both Organic and Inorganic Matter. (SP_{16})
Universal Intelligence gives force to both organic and inorganic matter.

CHAPTER 5

Editing the Universal Principles

Editing should be, especially in the case of old writers, a counseling rather than a collaborating task. The tendency of the writer-editor to collaborate is natural, but he should say to himself, "How can I help this writer to say it better in his own style?" and avoid "How can I show him how I would write it, if it were my piece?"

JAMES THURBER (1959)

The next step in exploring the metaphysical syllogism embedded in Stephenson's Thirty-Three Principles is to consider the structure of the principles themselves. In other words, we must ask ourselves what the words of these principles mean. Are they unambiguous and used consistently, clearly and grammatically? Are there any implicit assumptions that need to be made explicit, any archaic usages that might be updated for better clarity, or any grammatical constructions that could be improved? If so, how can we change them so that they say more clearly what Stephenson intended them to say?

Since our intent is to improve on Stephenson's original list of principles, not to replace them, editorial changes will need to be kept to a minimum. Those edits we do suggest here are the outcome of having taught, lectured on and discussed these principles with a long succession of classes full of inquiring chiropractic students, as well as numerous other chiropractic philosophers and practitioners over the course of the last twenty five years. As a result, a compelling deductive rationale for each and every suggestion is probably not necessary. Some of them are justified simply by familiarity of usage over the course of time. However, in all cases where an editorial change might be construed to alter the meaning or intent of the principle, the logic behind the suggestion will be provided.

Principle 1 Revised:

The first principle to consider in an altered form from Stephenson's original formulation is Principle 1, the Major Premise itself. Stephenson's Major Premise reads, *"A Universal Intelligence is in all matter and continually gives to it all its properties and actions, thus maintaining it in existence."* For the purpose of creating a well-structured "universal syllogism," this statement becomes: ***"There is a universal intelligence in all matter, continuously giving to it all its properties and*** *actions, thus maintaining it in existence, **and giving this intelligence its expression.**"* The rationale for each change is as follows.

Changing the subjective clause from "A Universal Intelligence is . . ." to "There is a universal intelligence . . ." actually entails two changes, both of which have the same purpose. By using "Universal Intelligence" as the active voice subject of the sentence, and by capitalizing it as a proper noun, Stephenson creates the perception that the concept of a "universal intelligence" necessarily implies a thing, or, more potentially confusingly, a "Being." In fact, the argument over whether the inclusion of "universal intelligence" in Chiropractic's Major Premise necessarily refers to or implies a belief in a "Supreme Being" or "God" has been controversial since the earliest writings of D. D. Palmer and B. J. Palmer explored the possible spiritual and religious implications of their own emerging health care beliefs.

This does not mean that the concept of a "universal intelligence" in the Major Premise is contradictory to a belief in God; rather it demands that we recognize that, as a naturalistic assumption, it is simply not the same thing as a belief in God.

On the other hand, our unique understanding of and interactions with human beings, in health and *dis-ease,*[11] is based on *natural laws.* ("Chiropractic is a philosophy, science and art of things natural...").[12] If so, this necessarily requires one to distinguish the concept of "universal intelligence" from one's belief (or *non*-belief) in the existence of a *meta-natural*[13] Supreme Being or God. This does not mean that the concept of a "universal intelligence" in the Major Premise is contradictory to a belief in God; rather it demands that we recognize that, as a naturalistic assumption, it is simply not the same thing as a belief in God. Consequently, to discourage the temptation to equate the term "universal intelligence" with belief in God from the very beginning, the term will be used without capitalization and in the passive voice (*There is a* universal intelligence), both in the Major Premise and throughout the syllogism.

The word "continually" is replaced with the word "continuously" simply because, while the term "continually" means "recurring regularly or frequently," it does not necessarily imply that the continual process is uninterrupted. (I have seen the sun rise in the morning *continually* throughout my life.) On the other hand, the term "continuously" does imply "uninterrupted." (I have experienced the pull of gravity *continuously* throughout my life.)[14] Since the subsequent development of the concept of the expression of a "universal intelligence" makes it

---

[11] *dis-ease:* the traditional chiropractic term for the lessening or loss of health *(ease)* through the incoordination of function and/or adaptation caused by interference to the transmission of internal, biological forces

[12] Stephenson's *Chiropractic Textbook,* p. *xiii*

[13] *meta-natural:* existing beyond the scope of natural law and outside of natural phenomena

[14] *Webster's New Universal Unabridged Dictionary,* Second Edition, p. 395-396

abundantly clear that universal intelligence's action on matter, via force, in over-coming the natural inertial passivity of matter, is continuous and uninterrupted (although distortable by interference), *continuously* is clearly the more correct term.

The last change is the most obvious and dramatic. It entails the addition of the clause *"and giving this intelligence its expression"* at the end of the principle. To the traditionalist reader, it may seem that an addition has been made to the Major Premise, thus necessarily altering its meaning. In fact, the situation is exactly op-posite this. With the addition of this clause, we recognize and make explicit an unvoiced, implicit assumption hiding within Stephenson's original premise.

Actually, this is a crucial addition. Without it, the Major Premise is an un-balanced assumption. As Stephenson wrote it, the Major Premise clearly estab-lishes the proposition of a fundamental duality existing at the heart of the universe's existence. This duality is very much the primary subject of chiropractic's metaphysical model. It is a true duality, not in the commonly held misperception of a duality as two opposite things existing in contention with each other, but in the more accurate sense of a "two-sided" nature to the existence of a single thing. In this conception, it is not unlike the duality of matter and energy. While matter and energy are commonly seen as representing two separate spheres of existence, differing from each other in clearly identifiable and describable ways, Albert Ein-stein, in his famous equation, $E = mc^2$, actually stated simply that energy and matter are just two different and interchangeable manifestations of the same fun-damental thing, namely "physical substance." The "duality" of matter and energy that lies at the heart of physical existence actually only describes the two poles of differentiation within the *unity* of substance.

Similarly, the fundamental "duality" implied in the Major Premise is actually just a description of the two "poles of differentiation" of a single "thing," which will be referred to as the "unity of all (natural) existence." This duality is actually more fundamental to existence than the duality of matter and energy, simply because the physical unity of all interacting matter and energy throughout the entire universe, i.e. the "substance" of the universe, forms only one aspect of the "duality" of existence. The other aspect of existence assumed in the Major Prem-ise is the "immaterial" aspect of existence, namely "intelligence," which forms the opposite "pole of differentiation" from the physical substance of the universe.

All of this is implied in the assumption of "a universal intelligence in all matter (substance)" and elaborated further in the brief description of the rela-tionship between intelligence and matter contained in the clause ". . . continu-ously giving to it (intelligence gives to matter) all its properties and actions . . ." However, the Major Premise stops short of defining the *interdependence* of both aspects of the duality, which is the fundamental nature of any true duality. In the basic physical duality of matter/energy, matter needs energy to give it motion, and energy needs matter to have something to move. In the material/immaterial duality, matter needs intelligence to give it its organization (properties and actions) and intelligence needs matter to . . . what? This is what is implied, but not stated in Stephenson's Major Premise, namely the other half of the relationship between intelligence and matter inherent in the duality.

The Major Premise tells us explicitly that immaterial intelligence gives physical matter its properties and actions (its organization). But it fails to state what physical matter gives to immaterial intelligence, which is equally essential to the duality. What matter gives to intelligence is, of course, the physical substrate necessary for the manifestation of intelligence's "intent to organize," which results in the "expression" of intelligence through the ongoing, dynamic evolution of matter's organization. This half of the assumption *must* be present in the Major Premise to give it internal integrity. Just as we are assuming that matter actually *exists* because of the properties and actions universal intelligence endows it with *("thus maintaining it* (matter) *in existence"),* we are also assuming that this "universal intelligence" *exists* because of its relationship with the material substance through which it expresses itself *("There is a universal intelligence **in all matter**. . . ").*

The concept of a universal intelligence, creative and potent with the possibilities of action, organization, interrelationship and form, but eternally frustrated by the absence of any medium (physical substance) upon which to act and through which to express its own eternal, creative potency, is not the universal intelligence assumed to exist in the Major Premise. In fact, the question of the existence of "intelligence" in the absence of any medium through which it can act and by which its existence might be known, is a meaningless question. It is only *in relationship to* the substance through which it is expressed, that the universal intelligence assumed in the Major Premise can even be said to actually exist. This is the dualistic symmetry that the addition of the final clause *"and giving this intelligence its expression"* explicitly creates.

Principle 2 Revised:

The only alteration made in Principle 2 (SP$_{17}$) is to change *"Every effect has a cause . . ."* to *"Every effect has **causes** . . ."* While this may appear to be a subtle change, it is necessary both to more correctly capture the concept of causality as we understand it today, and to bring the first clause of the principle into logical consistency with the formulation of the second clause of the original principle, *". . . and every cause has effects."*

Cause and effect both have to do with our assumption of the *temporal connectedness* of the present organizational state of the universe (its specific state of interrelatedness) to its future state of organization *(cause)*, and of the past organizational state of the universe to its present state of organization *(effects)*. Any "cause" or "effect" we care to consider is necessarily an artificial designation made relative to the single point in time and/or space at which we chose to examine the web of connectedness that leads up to that point, in the case of an effect, or forward from that point, in the case of a cause. Thus, just as *"every cause has effects"* gives recognition to the web-like, rather than linear, connectedness of reality, as we are beginning to understand it today, so *"every effect has causes"* does the same in considering any point's temporal connectedness to the universe's past. As reworded, this principle assumes the existence of web-like networks of interactive causes and effects, rather than reinforcing the more narrow and archaic view of cause and effect relationships as strictly linear chains of single, sequentially-connected events.

> **"Every cause has effects"** gives recognition to the web-like, rather than linear, connectedness of reality.

Principle 3 Revised:

Principle 3 – The Principle of Time (SP_6) is one of Stephenson's most well-known and oft quoted principles. As such, one might wonder why a change is necessary. What it says is clear and unambiguous, but there is no explanation offered or reason afforded as to why it should be phrased in the double negative *(There is **no** process that does **not** require time)*. Thus, for the purpose of grammatical parsimony and to eliminate the use of a double negative which doesn't seem to contribute anything to the validity or meaning of this basic assumption, it has been recast into its precisely equivalent positive form, *"All processes require time."*

Principle 4 Revised:

Principle 4 (SP_{15}) states that *"Matter can have no motion without the application of force by intelligence."* In reworking the syllogism, this principle will ultimately need to be changed slightly to read *"Matter can have no **organization** without the application of force by intelligence."* The need for this alteration is driven and justified by the changes already made to Principle 5 (see above) and further changes to be made in it (Principle 5) below. In Stephenson's *Chiropractic Textbook*, Principle 5 (SP_{14}) is called "Universal Life," which is also the topic it purports to illuminate. However, as discussed previously, the use of the term "life" in the concept of "universal life" is somewhat confusing and inconsistent with its use later in the principles specifically to denote the characteristics of biological life, vis-à-vis the common usage of the term. Closer examination of the principle suggests that the concept to which "universal life" refers is the *organization* created throughout the universe at all levels of existence by the action of intelligence. It is this use of the concept of *organization,* as the expression of *intelligence* in matter through the action of force, which needs to be captured in this principle.

As it stands, this principle (Principle 4) is composed of two parts; an assumption (specifically the assumption of the fundamental *inertial* property of matter), and a conclusion derived from the logical interaction between the first principle (the Major Premise) and the assumption of matter's essential inertia. The first part of this principle, *"Matter can have no motion without the application of force,"* is essentially Isaac Newton's First Law of Motion.

Newton's FIRST LAW OF MOTION

"Every object persists in its state of rest or uniform motion in a straight line unless it is compelled to change that state by forces impressed on it."

Newton stated this assumption as *"Every object persists in its state of rest or uniform motion in a straight line unless it is compelled to change that state by forces impressed on it."*[15] In terms of its use in this chiropractic syllogism, what this assumes is that matter, one of the forms of substance (the other being energy), is *passive.* Without an external influence, any material object, from an electron or proton to a galaxy, will simply continue to do what it is already doing, whether resting or moving, without responding to the actions of anything else around it. It is *inertial* (unresponsive) to any other matter, forming no relationships and participating in no *organizational interactions* unless acted on by an outside force. Under the influence of an outside force, matter's passivity can be overcome and its motion can begin, or be altered, *in response to that force.* Matter's response to force is to move or change its motion. This is the meaning of the first part of this principle as stated in Stephenson's original formulation.

However, the addition of the words *"Matter can have no motion without the application of force **by intelligence**"* changes everything. First, we have to ask why Stephenson added this qualification to the most basic of Newton's well-accepted Laws of Motion. The answer is logically obvious. Given that his *first principle* (the Major Premise) is the *assumption* that the organization of the universe (as embodied by the "properties and actions of matter") is caused by intelligence, the conclusion is inescapable that, since matter can have no motion without the action of force, it is the intelligence of the universe (the organizer) that must be the source of the universe's organizing forces.

The problem with this conclusion is that the concept that matter can have no *motion* without intelligent influence is not supported by the concept of what intelligence does. An action or a response is not "intelligent" just because it causes

---

[15] Isaac Newton's *Philosophiae Naturalis Principia Mathematica,* 1687

or changes the motion of some matter somewhere. Rather it is said to be "intelligent" if it changes matter's motion in some specific way that forms the meaningful, coordinated interactions between material parts that we name and describe as the "organization" of interrelated systems of matter *and energy,* producing an integrated whole *thing* (see Principle 6 below). In other words, force alone is sufficient to give passive matter the simple property of motion, but it takes *intelligence directing force* to give matter the complex interactions we call *organization.* It is the *organization* of matter *(how* it moves), and not just the mere fact of matter's motion *(that* it moves), which expresses and reveals the universe's inherent intelligence.

If this principle were applied only to the physical aspect of existence, it would read *"matter can have no motion without the application of force"* and stop there. And as such, it would be complete. But the philosophical conclusion which emerges from this purely physical principle, when interpreted in light of our primary assumption of the dual, material *and* immaterial nature of the universe, must read *"Matter can have no **organization** without the application of force **by intelligence.**"* In other words, the Major Premise assumes that the universe's "intelligence" is the *organizer* of matter, not just its *mover.*

Principle 5 Revised:

The reworking of Principle 4 (above) clarifies an issue first raised in relationship to the meaning of Principle 5 in our discussion of the rearrangement of Stephenson's Principles. In that discussion, it was noted that Principle 5 (SP_{14}), although Stephenson titled it "Universal *Life,*" actually referred to the action of a universal intelligence on *all* matter. It was further suggested that the term "life" in this principle should be exchanged for the more general term "organization," to maintain the distinction between universal principles of intelligent organization, in which group this principle clearly belongs, and the more specific principles concerning the intelligent organization of biological life. With this change, this principle becomes, *"Force is manifested by motion in matter; all matter has motion, therefore there is universal organization in all matter."*

In discussing the revisions to Principle 4 above, the case was made that force isn't just "manifested by *motion*" in matter, but that, in an intelligent, material/immaterial duality, **force, *as directed by a universal intelligence*, is manifested as *organization* in matter.** Thus, in considering the content and meaning of this principle, we must necessarily apply the same conclusion to it. This requires changing the wording of this principle in several places. *"Force is manifested by motion in matter;"* becomes *"Force is manifested **as organization** in matter;"* and *"all matter has motion,"* becomes *"all matter has **organization**,"*

Consequently, when we consider the conclusion the principle comes to, *"there-fore there is universal life* (as Stephenson put it) or *organization* (our first suggested revision) *in all matter,"* we realize that this is redundant with the new meaning of the first two clauses. What this principle should actually conclude is that there is **universal intelligence *expressed*** in all matter by its *current state of organization.*

With these changes, and a new title ("Universal *Expression"* rather than "Universal Organization" (Koch (above)) or "Universal Life" (Stephenson)) reflective of its clarified meaning, we discover that this principle is the pivotal conclusion derived from the assumptions inherent in the first five principles: *Force is manifested as organization in matter; all matter has organization, therefore there is universal intelligence expressed in all matter.* This conclusion parallels the Major Premise *(There is universal intelligence in all matter . . .)* but folds in the con-cept that it is *force,* acting on matter everywhere throughout the universe, which enables immaterial intelligence to organize physical matter. It is this con-clusion, placing *force* at the "interface" between the material and the immaterial, that lays the groundwork for our consideration and appreciation of the roles played by both *energy* (physical) and *information* (immaterial) in this dualistic interaction between the creative *(intelligence)* and the receptive *(matter),* which we know as existence.

Principle 6 Revised:

Principle 6 (SP_4) is a summative statement that codifies the central conclu-sion of the dualistic interactionalism slowly emerging out of Stephenson's Prin-ciples. In its current form it says, *"Organization* (rather than "Life" (see above)) *is a triunity having three necessary united factors, namely Intelligence, Force and Matter.* The only changes that may be useful to make in the wording of this summation involve a shift in emphasis as to what the "thing" to which this principle refers actually is. In its current form, *organization* is a property, whereas *Intelligence, Force* and *Matter* (notice again the capitalization characteristic of proper nouns) are either intended to denote or, at the very least, can be misinterpreted to denote the "things" referred to in this principle. The use of the term "triunity" reinforces this impression, implying three "things" interacting. This impression is further reinforced by the use of the construction *"having **three** necessary **united** factors"* which could logically lead us to ask the question, "If Intelligence, Force and Matter are the three factors united in "organization," what fourth "factor" must necessarily exist to unite these three?"

Our conceptualization of existence begins with an assumption (the Major Premise) that proposes a duality, not a triunity, as the core structure. And the "thing" being conceptualized is the intelligently organized universe itself, as a whole, or any portion of it (an atom, a living organism or a star). Intelligence, forces and matter are only *aspects* of the "thing we are describing" (existence itself), and *not* separate, individual "things" themselves. To illustrate; if we wish to conceptualize the existence of the "thing" called a marriage, we can begin with the assumption that it is fundamentally a dualistic structure, composed of male and female aspects, namely a man and a woman, who are different from each other, and both of whom play different, necessary and mutually complementary roles in the formation of the marriage *per se*. But to fully understand how a marriage can exist as a single, unified thing, we must also posit the existence of an additional factor involved in creating the dual nature of the marriage. This is, of course, the interactions between the two "parts;" the communications, shared experiences, common values, mutual consideration and affection; in short, the dynamic relationship between the dual aspects that creates the wholeness of the "thing *per se*," i.e. the marriage. Whereas this part of the whole thing (the *relationship*) can be named, it does not constitute a separate "thing *per se*" because the only "substance" of its existence is the actions of the two parts of the duality, the man and the woman. It has no existence separate from those actions.

Of course, this illustration is also an imperfect metaphor for our assumed "intelligence/ matter" duality, simply because, unlike a marriage, which *can* be dissolved by divorce (separation of the two partners), intelligence *cannot* exist independent of its expression through matter, any more than matter can exist without intelligent direction. The material/immaterial "marriage" assumed in the Major Premise cannot become "divorced," although it *can* suffer communication break-down, as we will see later.

To better identify the "thing" and the aspects of that "thing" to which this principle refers, it is proposed that we reword it to read *"Any organized structure is a triunity having three necessary factors, namely intelligence, matter and the force **which unites them.**"*[16] Note that the "thing *per se*" of this principle becomes that which exists (the universe as a whole or any organized structure which exists within it), the "aspects" of which are identified as "intelligence" and "matter," and the relationship between these aspects is identified and characterized by the "force which unites them." Because one aspect of this duality is physical (matter) and the other is immaterial (intelligence), force itself, which is the relationship between them, must not be a third new "thing" or "aspect" of existence. Rather, force is the *interface* between the material and the immaterial. As such, it must have both physical

> **Force is the interface between the material and the immaterial. As such, it must have both physical and immaterial aspects simultaneously.**

[16]My special thanks to Dr. Reggie Gold for his contribution to this rewording.

and immaterial aspects simultaneously, which we will find are embodied in the concepts of the *physical energy* and the *immaterial information* inherent in any organizing interaction.

These changes reveal an interesting new facet of the duality we are discussing. Although this duality in the Major Premise refers explicitly to the whole universe, it can also refer to any part of the whole. We can correctly conclude that *"any organized structure"* would refer to the universe as a whole, or any portion of it we care to consider, from a single proton, neutron or electron to an atom, a molecule, a living organism, the biosphere it is a part of, the planet it inhabits, the solar system, or even the galaxy which, of course, is a part of the universe as a whole. In this sense, this principle illustrates the distinctly "holographic" character of the Major Premise. Recollect that a *holograph* is an image storage matrix which, when illuminated by a laser light source similar to the one used to create it, produces a very precisely detailed, three dimensional image of the object that has been "holographed." The most interesting thing about a holograph is that, if you divide it in half, and illuminate either of the resulting halves of the holograph with a laser light source, you will get the whole image, although slightly less well-defined, rather than half of the original image. Divide that half-of-a-holograph again and illuminate any quarter of the original holograph, and you still get the entire image. In fact, *any portion* of the hologram will produce the whole image, at varying levels of distinctness proportional to the amount of the holograph being illuminated!

This is similar to the concept of the expression of intelligence through matter. If we could look at all the matter in the universe at one time, we would perceive and appreciate the complete expression of universal intelligence in perfect clarity at that moment in time. However, if we observe universal intelligence's expression through *any finite portion* of the universe's matter, we don't see the expression of just a small portion of universal intelligence; rather we see the complete expression of universal intelligence but with more or less clarity depending on the relative amount of matter we are considering. For example, a molecule possesses greater organizational complexity than any of the individual atoms of which it is composed. In fact, we recognize that the organizational complexity of each and every atom *is included* within the molecule, together with the greater organizational complexity of the molecule as a whole. But this doesn't mean that a molecule express *more* universal intelligence than an atom. Universal intelligence is *immaterial,* and, as such, there cannot be *more* or *less* of it, because "more" and "less" are physical concepts that simply do not apply to the immaterial. Rather, a molecule expresses universal intelligence *more clearly and completely* than it can be expressed in any one atom alone. If matter is universal intelligence's holograph, then when universal intelligence "illuminates" any portion of the universe's matter, it creates an image of universal intelligence's creativity proportional to the matter's ability to express organization and complexity. Ultimately, it will take all of the substance of the whole universe the entire span of its existence to fully express the creativity and complexity of form that exists as potential within the intelligence of the whole universe.

> **Ultimately, it will take all of the substance of the whole universe the entire span of its existence to fully express the creativity and complexity of form that exists as potential within the intelligence of the whole universe.**

Principles 7–10:

Principles 7, 8, 9 and 10 appear clear and logically consistent, without the need of any clarification or suggested revisions.

Principle 11 Revised:

The next principle that might be clarified, and thus improved, with some slight modification is Principle 11 (SP_{11}), which states in Stephenson's version, *"The forces of Universal Intelligence are manifested by physical laws; are unswerving and unadapted, and have no solitude for the structures in which they work."* There are only two minor revisions proposed. First, in addition to the decapitalization of "universal intelligence" suggested above, it is also helpful if we rearrange the subject slightly to read, *"The forces **the universe's intelligence creates** . . ."* Secondly, the use of the construction *"are manifested **by** physical laws"* implies that "physical laws" are some new element (some new and different "things" in and of themselves) introduced into Stephenson's syllogism. In actuality, the meaning of this principle is that the universally consistent matter/energy interaction that we, because of their very consistency, designate as the universes "physical laws" (e.g. gravitational attraction, electromagnetic interactions, Newton's Three Laws of Motions, quantum wave mechanics, etc.) are nothing more or less than the manifestation *of these universal forces,* which the universe's intelligence continuously creates and which the universe's matter continuously expresses. To better capture this meaning within the principle itself, we simply need to change the wording to say that universal forces are manifested **as** physical laws, rather than manifested **by** physical laws. Making these two subtle alterations produces a clearer, more polished version of this principle, which now reads *"The forces **the universe's intelligence creates throughout the universe** are manifested **as** physical laws; are unswerving and unadapted, and have no solicitude for the structures in which they work."*

Principles 12 and 13:

Like Principles 7–10 above, Principles 12 and 13 appear to require no clarifications or revisions.

Principle 14 Revised:

Finally, in Principle 14 (SP$_{16}$), the last of our Universal Principles, we need only to decapitalize "universal intelligence" to be consistent with the rest. It then becomes *"Universal intelligence gives force to both organic and inorganic matter."*

THE UNIVERSAL PRINCIPLES REARRANGED AND EDITED:

Making these changes, both substantial and editorial, to Stephenson's universal principles produces a "cleaned up" version of the logical syllogism that was dimly evident in the original list. Again, in order to maintain the continuity of this reinterpretation with Stephenson's original work, changes made to Stephenson's original formulations of these principles are identified by *italic* font.

No. 1. The Major Premise. (SP$_1$)
There is a universal intelligence in all matter, *continuously* giving to it all its properties and actions, thus maintaining it in existence, *and giving this intelligence its expression.*

No. 2. Cause and Effect. (SP$_{17}$)
Every effect has *causes* and every cause has effects.

No. 3. The Principle of Time. (SP$_6$)
All physical processes require time.

No. 4. No *Organization* without the Effort of Force. (SP$_{15}$)
Matter can have no *organization* without the application of force by intelligence.

No. 5. Universal *Expression.* (SP$_{14}$)
Force is manifested *as organization* in matter; all matter has *organization,* therefore there is universal *intelligence expressed* in all matter.

No. 6. The Triune of *Organization.* (SP$_4$)
Any organized structure is a triunity having three necessary factors, namely, intelligence, *matter and the force which unites them.*

No. 7. The Function of Intelligence. (SP$_8$)
The function of intelligence is to create force.

No. 8. The Amount of Intelligence in Matter. (SP$_7$)
The amount of intelligence for any given amount of matter is 100%, and is always proportional to its requirements.

No. 9. The Function of Force. (SP$_{10}$)
The function of force is to unite intelligence and matter.

No. 10. The Amount of Force Created by Intelligence. (SP$_9$)
The amount of force created by intelligence is always 100%.

No. 11. The Character of Universal Forces. (SP$_{11}$)
The forces *the universe's intelligence creates throughout the universe* are manifested *as* physical laws; are unswerving and unadapted, and have no solitude for the structures in which they work.

No. 12. Interference with Transmission of Universal Forces. (SP$_{12}$)
There can be interference with *the* transmission of universal forces.

No. 13. The Function of Matter. (SP$_{13}$)
The function of matter is to express force.

No. 14. Intelligence in Both Organic and Inorganic Matter. (SP$_{16}$)
Universal *i*ntelligence gives force to both organic and inorganic matter.

CHAPTER 6

The "Biological Principles"

We Chiropractors work with the subtle substance of the soul. . . . In the dim, dark, distant long ago, when the sun first bowed to the morning star, this power spoke and there was life; it quickened the slime of the sea and the dust of the earth and drove the cell to union with its fellows in countless living forms. Through eons of time it finned the fish and winged the bird and fanged the beast. Endlessly it worked, evolving its forms until it produced the crowning glory of them all. With tireless energy it blows the bubble of each individual life and then silently, relentlessly dissolves the form, and absorbs the spirit into itself again.

B. J. PALMER (1949)

Separating out the *universal principles* from Stephenson's Thirty-Three Principles leaves us with nineteen remaining principles that specifically address the issue of biological life. In Stephenson's original order and form, these are:

No. 2. The Chiropractic Meaning of Life.
The expression of this intelligence through matter is the Chiropractic meaning of life.

No. 3. The Union of Intelligence and Matter.
Life is necessarily the union of intelligence and matter.

No. 5. The Perfection of the Triune.
In order to have 100% Life, there must be 100% Intelligence, 100% Force, 100% Matter.

No. 18. Evidence of Life.
The signs of life are evidence of the intelligence of life.

No. 19. Organic Matter.
The material of the body of a "living thing" is organized matter.

No. 20. Innate Intelligence.
A "living thing" has an inborn intelligence within its body, called Innate Intelligence.

No. 21. **The Mission of Innate Intelligence.**
The mission of Innate Intelligence is to maintain the material of the body of a "living thing" in active organization.

No. 22. **The Amount of Innate Intelligence.**
There is 100% of Innate Intelligence in every "living thing," the requisite amount, proportional to its organization.

No. 23. **The Function of Innate Intelligence.**
The function of Innate Intelligence is to adapt universal forces and matter for use in the body, so that all parts of the body will have co-ordinated action for mutual benefit.

No. 24. **The Limits of Adaptation.**
Innate Intelligence adapts forces and matter for the body as long as it can do so without breaking a universal law, or Innate Intelligence is limited by the limitations of matter.

No. 25. **The Character of Innate Forces.**
The forces of Innate Intelligence never injure or destroy the structures in which they work.

No. 26. **Comparison of Universal and Innate Forces.**
In order to carry on the universal cycle of life, Universal forces are destructive, and Innate forces constructive, as regards structural matter.

No. 27. **The Normality of Innate Intelligence.**
Innate Intelligence is always normal and its function is always normal.

No. 28. **The Conductors of Innate Forces.**
The forces of Innate Intelligence operate through or over the nervous system in animal bodies.

No. 29. **Interference with Transmission of Innate Forces.**
There can be interference with the transmission of Innate forces.

No. 30. **The Causes of Dis-ease.**
Interference with the transmission of Innate forces causes incoordination of dis-ease.

No. 31. **Subluxations.**
Interference with transmission in the body is always directly or indirectly due to subluxations in the spinal column.

No. 32. **The Principle of Coordination.**
     Coordination is the principle of harmonious action of all the parts of
     an organism, in fulfilling their offices and purposes.

No. 33. **The Law of Demand and Supply.**
     The Law of Demand and Supply is existent in the body in its ideal
     state; wherein the "clearing house" is the brain, Innate the virtuous
     "banker," brain cells "clerks," and nerve cells "messengers."

Categorizing the Remaining Principles:

     In reviewing the remaining principles, one more categorization issue rele-
vant to our analysis of these principles as a logical syllogism becomes evident.
Most of these principles refer to the concepts involved with the interaction
between intelligence and matter within the body of a "living thing." This includes
any and every form of life, from single celled organisms (bacteria or protista) to
plants and animals to the living things chiropractic most directly concerns itself
with, namely human beings. Consequently, we will want to refer to these as the
"Biological Principles."

     However, a careful inspection will reveal that three of the remaining prin-
ciples address the intelligence/matter relationship in very *specific* biological
conditions, namely in living things with "nervous systems" and "spinal
columns." Consider SP_{28} (The Conductors of Innate Forces – *The forces of Innate
Intelligence operate through or over* **the nervous system** *in animal bodies.*), SP_{31} (Subluxations – *Interference with transmission in the body is always directly or indirectly due
to subluxations* **in the spinal column.**) and SP_{33} (The Law of Demand and Supply
– *The Law of Demand and Supply is existent in the body in its ideal state; wherein the
"clearing house" is* **the brain,** *Innate the virtuous "banker,"* **brain cells "clerks," and
nerve cells "messengers."**) In all three of these principles, the concepts of the whole
syllogism are applied specifically to issues of the transmission of forces to and
from the brain of an organism with a nerve system and a spinal column. This fact
distinguishes these three principles from the other sixteen. While the other sixteen
can presumably apply to any form of life, whether single- or multi-cellular,
whether plant or animal, these three apply specifically to vertebrates, and primarily to human beings. Clearly these are *more specific* than the title "biological
principles" implies. As such, these three principles suggest a third theme within
Stephenson's overall syllogism, and need to be separated out and placed into their
own category. With their relevance to the chiropractic profession's historic and
continuing focus on the clinical question of vertebral subluxation and its significance in human function and malfunction, it seems obvious that these constitute the only specifically "chiropractic" principles on the list. They will be referred

to as the "chiropractic principles" accordingly, and considered separately from the more general "biological principles" that precede them.

Segregating the three specifically chiropractic principles into their own category leaves us with sixteen biological principles. As with the universal principles above, it will again be useful to consider both the order of these principles and their specific content, to determine if we can arrange and edit them to create a stronger, clearer and more logically integrated form of this second "syllogism within the syllogism" of Stephenson's Principles.

CHAPTER 7

Rearranging the Biological Principles

Innate is the soul of the universe, concealed and revealed in an animal.

B. J. PALMER (1949)

Themdeletion of the three chiropractic-specific principles leaves Stephenson's Principles 2, 3, 5, 18–27, 29, 30 and 32. All of these principles address the nature of life, which we have interpreted above to refer specifically to biological life. First and foremost, these principles address the topic of life as a **subset** of the category of "all matter" established in the first principle *(There is a universal intelligence in **all matter** . . .)* This is evidenced by SP_{19} (Organic Matter), which states that *the material of the body of a "living thing" is organized matter.* It is this principle, therefore, that forms the logical segue into this portion of the syllogism. In defining the body of a living thing as "organized matter," this principle establishes that the following principles, concerning life and living things, are logically derived from Stephenson's universal principles, which address the larger issue of how intelligence organizes matter throughout the entire universe. Thus, with the assertion that life is a specific class of material organization, what must follow, and what does follow, is the logical model of how the principles of the intelligent organization of all matter apply specifically in the case of the intelligent organization of "living" matter. Therefore, in rearranging Stephenson's list of principles into a more coherent logical order, this principle (SP_{19}) necessarily becomes the first of the biological principles, now to be numbered Principle 15.

SP_{20}, the next principle in Stephenson's original listing, is actually the logical conclusion that follows naturally from the relationship between SP_{19} and the Major Premise. If the body of a living thing is organized matter (SP_{19}), and if there is a universal intelligence in *all* matter, continuously giving to it (all matter) all its properties and actions (Principle 1), in this case, its *living properties* (anatomy) and *living actions* (physiology), it must follow that this intelligence is also present in association with the organized matter of a living thing's body. Hence SP_{20} (Innate Intelligence) is precisely where it should be in relationship to our first biological principle. This, then, becomes our second biological principle, and is renamed Principle 16.

At this point, it becomes appropriate to reintroduce several of the principles we deleted earlier from the list of universal principles into our emerging list of biological principles. Both SP_2 (The Chiropractic Meaning of Life) and SP_3 (The Union of Intelligence and Matter) become logically sequential at this point in the syllogism, particularly since we are interpreting them as applying specifically to biological life. Thus SP_2 and SP_3 become Principles 17 and 18 in the emerging order of the biological principles. This positioning certainly clarifies their meaning, which was previously obscured by their original placement so early in the list, prior to the identification of life as a subset of universal organization.

Since Stephenson, in SP_2 (now our Principle 17), defines "life" as the expression of the intelligence of the universe through the matter of the body of a living thing, it becomes timely to note that the "signs of life"[17] referenced in SP_{18} (Evidence of Life) *constitute* the expression of this inborn intelligence of life. Logically, then, our next biological principle should be SP_{18}, which becomes Principle 19 in our new arrangement.

So far, we have rearranged the biological principles in this fashion: SP_{19}, SP_{20}, SP_2, SP_3, and SP_{18}. Next on Stephenson's list (if we continue to hold SP_5 (The Perfection of the Triune) for a later insertion at a more appropriate point in the developing syllogism) is SP_{21} (The Mission of Innate Intelligence – *The mission of Innate Intelligence is to maintain the material of the body of a "living thing" in active organization.*) Again, this principle constitutes the logical next step. Having identified and defined the innate intelligence of life, we can then distinguish its mission, as far as it is specific to the *living organization* of the matter of a living organism, from the more general "mission" of universal intelligence, which is to organize all matter generally. For this reason, SP_{21} becomes Principle 20 in our rearrangement.

With Principle 20 (SP_{21}) defining the mission of the living thing's innate intelligence, it follows that Principle 21 should then address *what is required* for the living thing's innate intelligence *to accomplish that mission* within the "living" matter through which it is expressing itself. This suggests that SP_5 (The Perfection of the Triune – *In order to have 100% Life, there must be 100% Intelligence, 100% Force, 100% Matter*) should be inserted into the syllogism here. Consequently, SP_5 becomes Principle 21.

The next two principles on Stephenson's list follow, in both number and order, the flow of the biological concepts in our current arrangement. Therefore, SP_{22} (The Amount of Innate Intelligence) and SP_{23} (The Function of Innate Intelligence) remain as Principles 22 and 23 in our new arrangement.

---

[17] Signs of life: those activities of a living thing which are considered to distinguishing "living organization" from other forms of organization, and specifically from the organization of the body that remains when life is no longer present, i.e. the corpse.

In reviewing these principles in their new order, we notice that Stephenson introduced an undefined concept in Principle 23 (The Function of Innate Intelligence – *The function of Innate Intelligence is to adapt universal forces and matter for use in the body, so that all parts of the body will have* **coordinated action** *for mutual benefit),* namely the concept of *coordination.* A quick look further down his list reveals that he does define it later, in his third to last principle, SP_{31} (The Principle of Coordination). Coordination, however, is so crucial a term at this point in the argument that it seems appropriate to move the later principle in which it is defined (SP_{31}) forward to follow Principle 23 directly. Thus, we will make SP_{31} our Principle 24, which causes SP_{24} (The Limits of Adaptation) to become our new Principle 25.

The next three of Stephenson's principles, SP_{25} (The Character of Innate Forces), SP_{26} (Comparison of Universal and Innate Forces) and SP_{27} (The Normality of Innate Intelligence) follow the logical flow and are in good order, with only one suggested rearrangement. In Stephenson's order, SP_{27} (The Normality of Innate Intelligence – *Innate Intelligence is always normal and its function is always normal),* which posits the *normality* of the living thing's innate intelligence and of its (innate intelligence's) function, and thus its beneficial and "constructive" effect on the body's state of organization, *follows* the two principles (SP_{25} and SP_{26}) that describe and characterize those internal forces as "constructive" and thus beneficial. Logically the principle that characterizes the actions of the living thing's innate intelligence *should precede* any principles that characterize the outcome/result of those actions. Rearranging these three principles accordingly again strengthens both the meaningfulness and the logical flow of the syllogism. Following this reasoning, the next three principles in our biological syllogism become Principle 26 – The Normality of Innate Intelligence (SP_{27}), Principle 27 – The Character of Innate Forces (SP_{25}), and Principle 28 – Comparison of Universal and Innate Forces (SP_{26}).

The function of Innate Intelligence is to adapt universal forces and matter for use in the body, so that all parts of the body will have *coordinated action* for mutual benefit.

Finally, having deleted SP_{28} (The Conductors of Innate Forces) for later consideration as a specifically chiropractic principle, we are left with SP_{29} (Interference with Transmission of Innate Forces), and SP_{30} (The Cause of *Dis-ease*). These principles now join our list, coincidentally in Stephenson's original number and order, as our Principles 29 and 30, and complete our categorization and rearrangement of Stephenson's biological principles.

We have now created a second subset of Stephenson's Principles, which we will list, as above, in their original wording but in the new order. Again, to avoid confusion and maintain the connection between Stephenson's first rough syllogism and this current work, the original order of each principle is indicated with an SP_n label, reflecting its earlier position. As before, following this listing, these principles will be subsequently referred to by their position in the new arrangement, rather than their position in Stephenson's original list, in order to take advantage of the logical strength of this rearrangement.

STEPHENSON'S "BIOLOGICAL PRINCIPLES" IN LOGICAL ORDER

No. 15. Organic Matter. (SP_{19})
The material of the body of a "living thing" is organized matter.

No. 16. Innate Intelligence. (SP_{20})
A "living thing" has an inborn intelligence within its body, called Innate Intelligence.

No. 17. The Chiropractic Meaning of Life. (SP_2)
The expression of this intelligence through matter is the Chiropractic meaning of life.

No. 18. The Union of Intelligence and Matter. (SP_3)
Life is necessarily the union of intelligence and matter.

No. 19. Evidence of Life. (SP_{18})
The signs of life are evidence of the intelligence of life.

No. 20. The Mission of Innate Intelligence. (SP_{21})
The mission of Innate Intelligence is to maintain the material of the body of a "living thing" in active organization.

No. 21. The Perfection of the Triune. (SP_5)
In order to have 100% Life, there must be 100% Intelligence, 100% Force, 100% Matter.

No. 22. The Amount of Innate Intelligence. (SP_{22})
There is 100% of Innate Intelligence in every "living thing," the requisite amount, proportional to its organization.

No. 23. The Function of Innate Intelligence. (SP_{23})
The function of Innate Intelligence is to adapt universal forces and matter for use in the body, so that all parts of the body will have coordinated action for mutual benefit.

No. 24. The Principle of Coordination. (SP_{32})
Coordination is the principle of harmonious action of all the parts of an organism, in fulfilling their offices and purposes.

No. 25. The Limits of Adaptation. (SP_{24})
Innate Intelligence adapts forces and matter for the body as long as it can do so without breaking a universal law, or Innate Intelligence is limited by the limitations of matter.

No. 26. The Normality of Innate Intelligence. (SP_{27})
Innate Intelligence is always normal and its function is always normal.

No. 27. The Character of Innate Forces. (SP_{25})
The forces of Innate Intelligence never injure or destroy the structures in which they work.

No. 28. Comparison of Universal and Innate Forces. (SP_{26})
In order to carry on the universal cycle of life, Universal forces are destructive, and Innate forces constructive, as regards structural matter.

No. 29. Interference with Transmission of Innate Forces. (SP_{29})
There can be interference with the transmission of Innate forces.

No. 30. The Causes of Dis-ease. (SP_{30})
Interference with the transmission of Innate forces causes incoordination of dis-ease.

CHAPTER 8

Editing the Biological Principles

Donald E. Carr points out that the sense impressions of one-celled animals are not edited for the brain: "This is philosophically interesting in a rather mournful way, since it means that only the simplest animals perceive the universe as it is."

ANNIE DILLARD (1998)

As we did with the universal principles above, it will again be useful to review and consider making appropriate changes to the wording and content of the biological principles. Continue to bear in mind that any changes suggested are intended to clarify the meaning and make the grammatical and logical structure of these principles more consistent, rather than to alter or deconstruct them in any way.

Principle 15:

Our first biological principle, Principle 15 (Organic Matter), is clear and concise in its original form and appears to require no revision.

Principle 16 Revised:

Our initial editorial suggestions involve Principle 16 (Innate Intelligence – *A "living thing" has an inborn intelligence within its body, called Innate Intelligence.)* There are two ways in which the wording of this principle is both confusing and inconsistent with our earlier work with the universal principles. The first confusing inconsistency lies in the usage of the phrase *". . . has an inborn intelligence within its body . . ."* At first glance, and in the absence of careful logical analysis, this wording has apparently suggested to many chiropractic students and philosophers that it introduces the concept of a new and different type of intelligence into our syllogism, namely the *innate intelligence* of life, as opposed to the *universal intelligence* of everything else (of atomic and molecular organization, of inorganic matter, of the dead body after life, of meta-organic matter (the planets, stars and galaxies that contain and sustain life). In fact, D. D. Palmer, in his earliest explorations of chiropractic's "philosophy of intelligence and matter" clearly refers to the "three intelligences" – Universal Intelligence, Innate Intelligence and Educated Intelligence.[18] Consequently, generations of chiropractors

[18] D. D. Palmer's *The Chiropractor's Adjuster*, p. 19 & 364

have perpetuated this misinterpretation of chiropractic philosophy in part because of the wording of this principle.

Furthermore, this misinterpretation has been exacerbated by the consistent misinterpretation of Principle 28 (Comparison of Universal and Innate Forces – *In order to carry on the universal cycle of life, Universal forces are destructive, and Innate forces constructive, as regards structural matter.*) Whereas this principle clearly characterizes universal *forces* as destructive, and innate *forces* as constructive, it is widely considered to characterize universal *intelligence* as destructive and innate *intelligence* as constructive, thus reinforcing the misimpression that they differ from each other, and represent two different intelligences at work in the same universe, one inside of living things and the other outside of living things.

The clear and inescapable inconsistency implicit in this interpretation of this principle, so strongly suggested by its problematic wording, is simply that the Major Premise, if it is to be accepted as our starting assumption, states that there is "a universal intelligence in *all matter* . . ." (an inescapably inclusive category that necessarily implies any and all "living matter" as well), ". . . continuously giving to it *(all* matter) *all its properties and actions* . . ." (an absolutely inclusive category that necessarily includes any and all "living properties" matter may express at any time anywhere in the universe). In other words, the intelligence to which this principle refers is not another type of intelligence than *universal intelligence,* nor it is a particular part, parcel or portion of *universal intelligence.* Rather it is simply *universal intelligence itself.* If *universal intelligence* gives *all* matter *all* its properties and actions, then it must give *living* matter all its *living* properties and actions. This concept, which Stephenson "called Innate Intelligence" in this principle, is just the *specific name* he is using *for universal intelligence* when it is being expressed by what we call "life."

Given the logical inconsistency between the Major Premise and the seemingly very common misinterpretation of this principle that implies a difference between the concepts of *universal intelligence* and *innate intelligence,* it is necessary to ask how this principle might be reworded to disallow such a misinterpretation and correct the resulting inconsistency. This is not as difficult as it might seem, given the magnitude of the confusion that exists over this issue. Rather than saying that a living thing ". . . **has** an inborn intelligence within its body, called its *Innate Intelligence,"* we need to simply be more explicit in stating that this principle is a direct deductive conclusion from the relationship between Principle 1 (The Major Premise – *There is a universal intelligence in all matter, continuously giving to it all its properties and actions, thus maintaining it in existence, and giving this intelligence its expression)* and Principle 15 (Organic Matter – *The material of the body of a "living thing" is organized matter).* If these two principles are true, then

Principle 16 needs only to say that a living thing has *the intelligence **of the universe** inborn within it*. And rather than calling it *Innate Intelligence* (notice again the archaic, personifying capitalization), let us refer to it here and throughout the rest of the syllogism as the *innate intelligence* (uncapitalized) of the living thing.

Finally, the quotation marks around the term "living thing" can be dropped in this and subsequent principles. These quotation marks first appear and are appropriate in Principle 15 (SP_{19}). As the first of our biological principles, Principle 15 introduces the concept that the biological principles specifically address the topic of "living things." After this, having solved the issue of Stephenson's ambiguous use of the term "life" by categorizing his principles more accurately as either universal and biological principles, there is no need to continue setting off the term *living thing* with quotation marks following its first introduction into the syllogism.

With these editorial changes, Principle 16 now states that *"A living thing has the intelligence of the universe inborn within it, referred to as its innate intelligence."*

Principle 17 Revised:

Principle 17 is titled the "Chiropractic Meaning of Life." It says *"the expression of this intelligence (innate intelligence as identified in Principle 16) through matter is the Chiropractic meaning of life."* In every respect except one, this appears to be clear and to follow logically from the universal principles and Principle 16. However one point of clarification in the phrase *"the Chiropractic **meaning of life**"* might be helpful. In this principle, Stephenson is clearly defining what the term "life" means, as deduced from his prior principles. In many other contexts, however, the phrase "the meaning of life" refers to the human search for the meaningfulness and purpose of one's existence and actions while alive. Nonetheless, nothing about this principle, or the subsequent philosophical concepts that flow from it, suggest that Stephenson intended this phrase to allow for such an interpretation. To clarify that Stephenson's meaning in this principle is nothing more or less than his philosophical *definition* of life, rather than a statement concerning its *meaningfulness,* quotation marks are placed around the term "life." Principle 17 (The Chiropractic Meaning of Life – *The expression of this innate intelligence through matter is the chiropractic[19] meaning of "life."*) now becomes unambiguously definitional, rather than possibly misinterpretable as a value judgment on the search for meaning to human life.

Principle 18 Revised:

What is now our Principle 18 (The Union of Intelligence and Matter – *Life is necessarily the union of intelligence and matter),* started out on Stephenson's list as

---

[19] Note the decapitalization of the adjective "chiropractic" in keeping with modern rules of capitalization.

Principle 3 (SP₃). As Stephenson's third principle, it was very confusing, simply because Stephenson started with a Major Premise about the whole universe, and followed immediately with two principles (The Chiropractic Meaning of Life and The Union of Intelligence and Matter) about the meaning and nature of "life." He went on, as we have noted in the universal principles above, to deduce the principle he named "The Triune of Life (Intelligence, Force and Matter), which we subsequently renamed the "Triune of Organization," as per the arguments presented above.

When we bring this principle into the biological principles, it becomes immediately obvious that, as a biological principle *per se,* it reintroduces the Triune of Organization into the issue of the nature of life. This principle needs only to have the concept of the role of force, as developed in the universal principles above, inserted into it. This addition will allow this principle to relate the Triune of Organization specifically to living things, and will transform it into a more correctly named "Triune of Life" than Stephenson's original, inappropriately named, universal principle (Principle 6 – The Triune of Organization (SP₄)).

If we add the concept of force as the "link" between intelligence and matter within a living thing, as the universal principles say it is in *all matter,* Principle 18 will now read *"Life is necessarily the union of **this** intelligence and **the matter** of a living thing, brought about by the creation of specific internal (innate) forces."*[20]

Principle 19 Revised:

We can improve Principle 19 (Evidence of Life – *The signs of life are evidence of the intelligence of life.)* with the simple addition of what the "signs of life" are. In his *Chiropractic Textbook,* Stephenson puts forth the list the five "abilities" (the ability to *assimilate, eliminate, grow, reproduce* and *adapt)*[21] that he believes all living things share, and which he thus considers distinctive to, and therefore definitive of, a living thing. Indeed, it would be a productive discussion to explore what the "signs of life" actually mean, and how this concept reinforces the idea that it is the expression of its own, organism-wide *innate intelligence* that both creates life and defines what it is. Nonetheless, for the purpose of clarifying and revising our biological principles to better work together as an integrated, logical syllogism, it is enough at this point to insert Stephenson's list of "the signs of life" into the principle, which will then read, *"The signs of life (the ability to assimilate, eliminate, grow, reproduce and adapt) are evidence of the intelligence of life."*

---

[20]Special thanks to Reggie Gold for his contributions to the specific wording of this principle.
[21]Stephenson's *Chiropractic Textbook,* Art. 334, p. 256

Principles 20–23 Revised:

Principles 20–23 need nothing more than the alterations in punctuation we have already made in the principles above. Principle 20 (The Mission of Innate Intelligence – *The mission of Innate Intelligence is to maintain the material of the body of a "living thing" in active organization.*) will now read, *"The mission of a living thing's innate intelligence is to maintain the material of its body in active organization."* Likewise, Principle 21 (The Perfection of the Triune – *In order to have 100% Life, there must be 100% Intelligence, 100% Force, 100% Matter.*) becomes *"In order to have 100% life, there must be 100% intelligence, 100% force, and 100% matter."* Principle 22 (The Amount of Innate Intelligence – *There is 100% of Innate Intelligence in every "living thing,".* . .) becomes *"There is 100% of innate intelligence in every living thing, the requisite amount, proportional to its organization."* And Principle 23 (The Function of Innate Intelligence – *The function of Innate Intelligence is . . .*) becomes *"The function of a living thing's innate intelligence is to adapt universal forces and matter for use in its body, so that all parts of its body will have coordinated action for mutual benefit."*

Principle 24 Revised:

Principle 24 (The Principle of Coordination – *Coordination is the principle of harmonious action of all the parts of an organism, in fulfilling their offices and purposes.*) presents a more subtle opportunity to reinforce the interactional nature of the model put forth in this syllogism, while at the same time clarifying the concept of the principle itself, by simply updating its terminology. It is strictly a definitional statement, presented to illuminate the concept of "coordinated action for mutual benefit" used in Principle 23 above. In fact, we moved Principle 24 forward from its original position as SP_{32} for the express purpose of providing the definition directly following the initial use of the concept.

We can now improve this definition by replacing the phrase *"harmonious action of all parts of an organism"* (what is a *harmonious action* in harmony with?) with the more grammatically correct phrase *harmonious **interaction** **among** all parts of an organism*. This may seem a small change, but it produces a large improvement in the clarity of this definition, which is now more consistent with the interactionalism of Principle 23.

Secondly, we might consider replacing the terms *offices* with the more familiar biological term *function* in the phrase *"in fulfilling their offices and purposes."* Within the body of the text itself, Stephenson describes the job that one part of the body (i.e. a tissue cell) fulfills, in meeting the needs of the body as a whole, as its *function*.[22] This is a much more traditional term for its biological role

---

[22] Stephenson's *Chiropractic Textbook*, Art. 82, p. 48

than its *office,* which has a more sociological, almost bureaucratic ring to it. With these changes in place, Principle 24 states, *"Coordination is the principle of harmonious interaction among all the parts of an organism, in fulfilling their functions and purposes."*

Principle 25 Revised:

Next we come upon Principle 25 (The Limits of Adaptation – *Innate Intelligence adapts forces and matter for the body as long as it can do so without breaking a universal law, or Innate Intelligence is limited by the limitations of matter.)* In terms of logical integrity, coming to this point in the syllogism is a little like driving over the top of a hill and suddenly coming up on a car wreck. You may be asking, "Why would the author say that?" Examine the final clause of Stephenson's principle closely. Consider it as a stand alone concept: *". . . Innate Intelligence is limited by the limitations of matter."* Surely this cannot be what Stephenson meant to say! How can the body's innate intelligence, which is *immaterial,* which is the intelligence of the universe, which is always 100%, always giving matter its properties and actions, and thereby giving *matter* its limits, . . . how can this innate intelligence *itself* be limited? . . . by anything?

Actually, this appears to be simply a logical slip that has stood uncorrected since Stephenson's *Chiropractic Textbook* was published in 1927, and was reprinted without revision, other than the addition of Galen Price's text on the *Occipito-Atlanto-Axial Region,* in 1948. In fact, Stephenson's metaphysical dualism does *not* propose limitations to intelligence *per se.* Rather, in every case where limitations are discussed, these are limitations of the *organization* that results from the *expression* of intelligence through matter, and not limits on intelligence itself. Organization, as an expression of the intelligence of a finite system, or of the universe as a whole, is physical and thus always has limits. In fact, limits, by their very definition, are physical (too much, not enough, the wrong quality). It is the *physical* properties of any particular state of organization that determine its nature and define its limits. Even as the organization of a thing changes, its properties change, and its limits change as well. But the intelligence which creates the organization isn't physical; therefore it doesn't change, even though it is expressed through physical changes, which are themselves organized (i.e. physical *processes)* and have their own limits.

Furthermore, since intelligence is immaterial, its existence *per se* can only be understood as encompassing the limitless field of *possibilities* which exists to be manifested as *reality* (actually a continuous unfolding of *realities* over time) through the process of the expression of *potential* organization *(thought* or *form)* as *actual* organization (material "parts" interacting in specific, therefore limiting, relationships). If *intelligence* can only be said to actually exist in the form of all the *possibilities of organization* inherent in all of existence, this "field of possibilities" cannot be limited by the matter through which it is being expressed, while at the same time being defined as that *unlimited potential* from which the organization of matter is created.

Of course, the solution to this logical conundrum is simple enough. It just requires that we reword the principle to better reflect the basic duality of the syllogism. It is the *physical expression* of innate intelligence that is limited by the limitations of matter (and *time,* as well, according to Principle 3), rather than innate intelligence *itself.* Thus our reworked Principle 25 will read, *"A living thing's innate intelligence adapts forces and matter for use in its body as long as it can do so without breaking a universal law; in other words, **its expression** is limited by the limitations of matter **and time.**"*

Principle 26 Revised:

Principle 26 (The Normality of Innate Intelligence – *Innate Intelligence is always normal and its function is always normal.)* presents no other problem than the decapitalization we have been using to reinforce the depersonification of the concept of intelligence throughout these principles. This principle will read more clearly as *"A living thing's innate intelligence is always normal and its function is always normal."* However, although it doesn't require any further modification, there is one other comment to make on the clarity of the wording of this principle, Where this principle says "and *its function* is always normal," *its function* refers to *innate intelligence's* function ("to adapt universal forces and matter for use in the body, so that all parts of the body will have coordinated action for mutual benefit" – Principle 23 above), not the physical functioning of the body itself. As we know from Principle 25 above, the functioning of the physical body, which is the *expression* of the innate intelligence's function (to adapt universal forces and matter for use in the body), **is** limited, by the limits of matter and time, and therefore may well *not* be "normal" even though the body's *innate intelligence* and *its* functioning is always "normal" by definition.

Principle 27 Revised:

Principle 27 (The Character of Innate Forces – *The forces of Innate Intelligence never injure or destroy the structures in which they work.)* presents several logical challenges that require some careful thought about what Stephenson intended this principle to mean, followed by some clarification in terminology to better capture that meaning. Appropriately decapitalized, the subject of this principle reads *"The forces **of a living thing's** innate intelligence . . ."* What is this actually supposed to mean? It can't mean the forces the living thing's innate intelligence *possesses.* A living thing's innate intelligence doesn't *have* any forces; in fact, it *can't have* any forces, because it is immaterial, whereas forces are (at least partially) material. Principles 23 and 25 (above) both say that a living thing's innate intelligence *adapts universal forces* (and matter) for use in the body. In doing so, we say that a living thing's innate intelligence *creates* new forces, specifically *innate (biological) forces,* out of the universal forces it adapts (changes) to be useful in meeting the body's specific needs. But a living thing's innate intelligence doesn't *have* these forces, the body itself, its physical structure, does. For a living thing's innate intelligence to *adapt* (change) a force, first the body must absorb it or take it in somehow. Then the living thing's innate intelligence must alter it somehow to be useful in meeting the body's physical needs. Even though a new *innate* (adapted) *force* is now carrying the constructive *information* the living thing's innate intelligence has endowed it with, which is *immaterial,* nonetheless the force itself is physical. In fact, it *must* be physical in order for it to be transmitted throughout the body, and in order for it to be able to cause the organizational/functional changes the living thing's innate intelligence created it to cause. Thus, rather than *"The forces of a living thing's innate intelligence . . .,"* the subject of this principle should say *"The forces a living thing's innate intelligence **creates** . . ."*

The rest of the principle then goes on to say that these forces a living thing's innate intelligence creates *never injure or destroy the structures in which they work.* This statement can be interpreted problematically in two different ways. The first problem arises with the concept of interference, which is introduced, relative to universal forces, in Principle 12 and which will be reintroduced, relative to "innate" forces, in Principle 29. According to both of these principles, once intelligence creates a force, that force is vulnerable to *interference,* and if it is interfered with, it can then go on to create *dis-*organization, rather than the organization intelligence *intended to cause* by creating the force in the first place. In terms of a living thing, this means that any force a living thing's innate intelligence creates, *if interfered with,* can in fact then injure or even destroy the very structures in which it works, namely the living thing's body itself. Of course, this also assumes that *interference* doesn't create a new force; rather it just alters and distorts a force which a living thing's *innate intelligence* actually created. And this is exactly what Stephenson concludes and codifies in Principle 30 (The Cause of Dis-ease) (see discussion below). Thus, we can say that an *innate force,* created by a living thing's innate intelligence to coordinate its body's actions, actually does, *if interfered with and distorted,* end up injuring or even destroying the structure in which it works, in direct contradiction to the principle itself. To eliminate such an interpretation of this principle, it is both more correct and more defensible to say that *the forces a living thing's innate intelligence creates **are never intended to** injure or destroy the structures in which they work.*

Even with the rewording above, however, there still exists a second possible interpretation of this principle that also contradicts it. This has to do with the fact that in any complex, internally inter-dependent, multi-cellular life form, the well-being of the component parts (structures) of the organism, namely its cells, is clearly *subjugated to the well-being of the whole organism.* Because of this, especially in cases of trauma or attack, a living thing's innate intelligence, with its *organism-wide* perspective, may well injure or even destroy some of the body's own structures in order to save or insure the survival of the organism as a whole.

For example, if a human being were to suffer a microbial invasion and send its macrophages into action to attack and kill the invading microbes, this response, *caused by* innate forces created by the body's own innate intelligence, may well serve the "good of the whole body," while still causing the deaths of many of the macrophages themselves, which are certainly human body cells. (Don't forget that every one of the macrophages that sacrifices itself for the survival of the organism as a whole is a genetic identical twin of every other cell in the body, and putatively has just as strong an innate vitality and will to live as every other one of its brother or sister cells.)

Another illustrative example occurs in cases of starvation. Deprived of food, many an organism will begin to digest and consume its own muscle tissue to provide the energy needed to keep other vital systems alive, perhaps long enough to find food and survive, against the hope that it will then be able to rebuild the destroyed muscle tissue. Thus, to survive, a living thing's innate intelligence most certainly intends to "injure or destroy the structures in which (its innate forces) work." Notice, however, that in these examples the living thing's innate intelligence is using the resources at hand to continue to express itself through the organism as a whole, even though some of those "resources" are a part of the body itself. This is *not* a contradiction of Principle 23 (The Function of Innate Intelligence – *The function of a living thing's innate intelligence is to adapt universal forces and matter for use in its body, so that all parts of its body will have coordinated action for mutual benefit.*) if we consider that some of the matter the living thing's innate intelligence must adapt is the matter of the body itself. Nor does it contradict Principle 24 (The Principle of Coordination – *Coordination is the principle of harmonious interaction among all the parts of an organism, in fulfilling their functions and purposes.*) if we consider that it is a living thing's innate intelligence itself that establishes the appropriate "functions and purposes" of all of the body's parts in the first place. If one of the functions of a tissue is to sacrifice itself for the good of the whole body, the living thing's innate intelligence *is* injuring or destroying some part of the organism to ensure the survival of, and thus its own expression through, the whole organism. This is actually a part of the very definition of the innate intelligence of a living thing, namely it is the consciousness of the needs of the whole, integrated organism, over and above the needs of its parts. Nonetheless, it would contradict this principle's claim that innate forces are **never** intended to injure or destroy any living structures in which they work. The final editorial change we can make to eliminate this internal contradiction is to say that *"The forces a living thing's innate intelligence creates are never intended to injure or destroy the **living thing itself."***

Principle 28 Revised:

The main challenges in Principle 28 (Comparison of Universal and Innate Forces – *In order to carry on the universal cycle of life, Universal forces are destructive, and Innate forces constructive, as regards structural matter.*) are all matters of the interpretation of how this principle is worded, rather than what it is trying to say. In my experience teaching these concepts, this is one of the most misinterpreted, and therefore misunderstood, of Stephenson's principles.

He refers to the two types of forces he is designating here as "Universal forces" and "Innate forces." The capitalizations he uses clearly indicate that he is naming these two different kinds of forces (one destructive, the other constructive) in terms of *which intelligence creates them.* "Universal forces" are those created by Universal Intelligence, the intelligence of the entire universe, whereas "Innate forces" are those created by Innate Intelligence, the intelligence of a living thing. But as we have explored earlier, a living thing's innate intelligence *is* universal intelligence, as it exists in the matter of the body.[23] Because of this, different kinds of forces *cannot be distinguished* by "which kind of intelligence" creates them; the universe's intelligence creates *all* of the forces in the entire universe, including those it creates by adapting external forces assimilated into the functioning bodies of living things. In fact, the actual distinction between a "universal force" and an "innate force" is not "what kind of intelligence" creates each "type" of force. Rather, it is *at what level of organization* intelligence creates a force that determines its "type."

When discussing the various types of forces acting upon and within *a specific living thing,* we can clearly distinguish two distinctly different categories of forces at play. All of the forces involved that the universe's intelligence creates which are not associated with the biological functioning of that specific living thing (forces created *externally* to it or at the atomic and molecular levels of its

---

[23] This is just another example of the confusion that arises from the use of personifying capitalizations.

own matter's organization) can be considered *environmental forces* (those forces that determine the *environment* within which the living organization must be created). At the same time, the forces the universe's intelligence creates in the process of *"adapting universal forces and matter for use in the body"* (in which case, we will designate the intelligence of the universe as the living thing's *innate intelligence)*, in other words, forces created *internally* through the physiological processes of life within that specific living thing itself, can be identified as *internal biological forces.*

With this interpretation of what "universal forces" and "innate forces" mean, it is important to note that *all* the forces being created continuously at the atomic and molecular levels of organization, even those within a living thing's matter, which the universe's intelligence creates in matter whether it is a part of a specific living thing's structure or not, would have to be classified as *environmental* (universal) forces. Thus, the forces that hold a water molecule together are *environmental* forces, whether that water molecule is within the ocean or within your circulatory system. On the other hand, the forces that *move* the ocean's currents are *environmental* forces, whereas the forces that move the blood through your circulatory system are your own *internal biological* (innate) *forces.* To capture this distinction between universal forces and innate forces, as defined relative to any specific living thing, it is suggested that we change "universal forces," when considered in relationship to a specific living organism, to *environmental forces,* and change "innate forces" to *internal biological forces,* wherever these terms are used throughout the principles.

> When discussing the various types of forces acting upon and within a specific living thing, we can clearly distinguish two distinctly different categories of forces at play. Thus, the forces that hold a water molecule together are *environmental forces,* whether that water molecule is within the ocean or within your circulatory system. On the other hand, the forces that move the ocean's currents are environmental forces, whereas the forces that move the blood through your circulatory system are your own *internal biological (innate) forces.*

Having clarified what Stephenson means by *universal forces* and *innate forces,* let us next address how he characterizes them. His principle says *". . . Universal forces are destructive, and Innate forces constructive, as regards structural matter."* Our rewording produces this result: *"In order to carry on the universal cycle of life, **environmental forces** are destructive, and **internal biological forces** are constructive, as regards structural matter."*

One problem that arises from Stephenson's characterization of environmental forces as patently destructive, without any qualification, is that it creates inherent confusion as to the role they play in adaptation and survival. To say that the food, water and oxygen we continuously assimilate from our environment, all of which are thus "environmental forces" acting on the body, "are destructive," seems to stand in contradiction to the fact that we clearly *need* these very forces, along with others, to survive. How can we need forces which are destructive, in order to survive? Does this principle mischaracterize such forces? Are some types of environmental forces destructive, while others are constructive? Or can any particular environmental force be either destructive or constructive, depending on the situation, and we must distinguish when an environmental force may be destructive, i.e. water in which we may drown, versus when it may be constructive, i.e. water which will satisfy our thirst?

Another difficulty that arises from Stephenson's unqualified characterization of environmental forces as destructive, is that it tends to lead many students of chiropractic philosophy to misinterpret this principle to mean that, since it creates environmental forces which are destructive, *universal intelligence* itself must *be destructive*. This also implies that *innate intelligence* is the *constructive intelligence* of life, working in opposition to universal intelligence's inherent destructiveness. In fact, this is a serious error in reasoning. First and foremost, universal intelligence is attributed to be the cause of all organization in the universe, including the organization of life itself, which is by definition constructive; and secondly, universal intelligence cannot be conceived of as working in opposition to a living thing's innate intelligence if both *universal intelligence* and *innate intelligence* are, in fact, just two different names for the same organizing intelligence.

The solution to the problems that arise from this absolute characterization of environmental forces as destructive, is to qualify it with the concept that it is the role of a living thing's *innate intelligence* to convert the potential destructiveness of the environmental forces that impact on the body into something that *is constructive* to the body, exactly as is proposed in Principle 23 (The Function of Innate Intelligence – *The function of a living thing's innate intelligence is to* **adapt** *universal forces and matter for use in its body, so that all parts of its body will have coordinated action for mutual benefit.)* Thus we will characterize environmental forces as (intrinsically) destructive, *unless they can be adapted* by the body's innate intelligence. In this case, they (the *adapted* environmental forces) *become* internal biological forces by being transformed from being intrinsically destructive to being intrinsically *constructive*.

The same problems which plague the unqualified characterization of environmental forces as destructive also apply to the unqualified characterization of internal biological forces as constructive. This would seem to imply that an "intrinsically constructive" biological force must always be beneficial and useful, and can never be harmful, to the body in which it is created. Yet the following two principles, Principle 29 (Interference with Transmission of Innate Forces – *There can be interference with the transmission of Innate forces.*) and Principle 30 (The Causes of Dis-ease – *Interference with the transmission of Innate forces causes incoordination of dis-ease.),* outline the very situation in which an internal biological force, which this principle characterizes as constructive, will cause incoordination *(dis-ease),* i.e. if it suffers interference. Thus, the very forces created by a living thing's innate intelligence to be constructive to the body become *destructive* forces as a consequence of interference (an alteration of the force during its transmission).

Again, the solution lies in the insertion of the appropriate qualification into the text of the principle. Internal biological forces should be characterized as constructive, *unless they suffer interference,* at which point the intrinsic constructive quality they are endowed with by the body's innate intelligence is altered, distorted and degraded to the point that they can cause *dis*-organization (inco-ordination or *dis-ease)* rather than the organization they were intended, and created, to cause (coordination, normal function and health).

The final editorial change proposed to strengthen and clarify this principle has to do with the use of the phrase *"as regards structural matter."* Clearly, the "structural matter" referred to is the physical substance of a living thing, specifically the living thing that is being subjected to the destructive character of any environmental forces which impinge on it, and/or the constructive character of the internal biological forces it is creating and expressing within itself. Rather than introducing a new term *(structural matter),* not used before in the syllogism, the clearest way to illustrate the difference between the forces being characterized and the matter in relationship to which they are being identified and defined, is to name it specifically in the case of each kind of force. Thus the principle as we have edited it so far – *In order to carry on the universal cycle of life, environmental forces are destructive, unless they can be adapted, whereas internal biological forces are constructive, unless they suffer interference, as regards structural matter* – would adopt its final form as *"In order to carry on the universal cycle of life, environmental forces are destructive to a specific living thing, unless it can adapt them, whereas internal biological forces are constructive to the specific living thing that creates them, unless they suffer interference."*

Finally, to apply these conclusions consistently, we will want to revisit any other biological principles that make reference to either "Universal forces" (Principle 23 above) or "Innate forces" (Principle 27 above, Principles 29 & 30 below) and substitute the terms "environmental forces" and "internal biological forces" respectively, for these more archaic terms.

Principles 29 & 30 Revised:

Both Principle 29 (Interference with Transmission of Innate Forces – *There can be interference with the transmission of Innate forces.)* and Principle 30 (The Causes of Dis-ease – *Interference with the transmission of Innate forces causes incoordination of dis-ease.)* are simple, straightforward and unambiguous. There are two small changes to make, however; one to be consistent with the reasoning we developed in consideration of the principle above, and the other to correct a typographical error that has caused confusion and misinterpretation for the last eighty-one years.

First, as reasoned above, we should change the name of the forces referred to in both of these principles from "Innate forces" to *internal biological forces.* Thus Principle 29 becomes *"There can be interference to the transmission of internal biological forces."* And Principle 30 reads *"Interference with the transmission of internal biological forces causes incoordination of dis-ease."*

Secondly, contemplating Principle 30, it appears that there is a grammatical error in the phrase "causes incoordination of dis-ease." It would appear that this would be more grammatically correct if it said, *"Interference . . . causes **the** incoordination of dis-ease."* However, this wording would strongly suggest that *incoordination* and *dis-ease* are two different concepts, with *incoordination* being a property of *dis-ease.* Saying *"the incoordination **of** dis-ease"* is like saying the color *of* my hair. In this construction, *color* is a property, and not necessarily the only property, of my hair. There is more to my hair than just its color. Likewise, this wording suggests that there is more to *dis-ease* than just the *incoordination of dis-ease.* However, in the textual usage of the terms *incoordination* and *dis-ease,* Stephenson emphasizes several times that *dis-ease* **is** *incoordination* and *incoordination* **is** *dis-ease.* He uses them synonymously.

This mystery is solved if we refer directly to the article in the Senior Text of Stephenson's *Chiropractic Textbook* that discusses this principle specifically. There we find this principle written as follows: "Interference with the transmission of Innate forces causes incoordination *or* (emphasis added) dis-ease."[24] In fact, there is no discrepancy between this principle as it is listed in the Thirty-Three Principles at the front of the book, and as it is discussed and developed in the text, just an eighty-one-year-old typographical error that has never been noticed, or corrected. It was faithfully reproduced in the 1948 edition of Stephenson's *Chiropractic Textbook,* which is still reproduced and sold today, and on innumerable charts and lists of the Thirty-Three Principles distributed by chiropractic

---

[24] Art. 364, p. 301

philosophy enthusiasts worldwide. But since this simple, innocent typo still has the potential to cause misinterpretation and confusion concerning the meaning of this principle, and especially the meaning of the terms *incoordination* and *dis-ease*, it is time to correct it. In order to be consistent with the overall logical syllogism, this principle should read *"Interference with the transmission of internal biological forces causes in-coordination, **or** dis-ease."* This appears to be how Stephenson intended it to be worded in the first place.

... just an eighty-one-year-old typographical error that has never been noticed, or corrected.

STEPHENSON'S BIOLOGICAL PRINCIPLES REARRANGED AND EDITED

We have completed our reevaluation, editing and reworking of Stephenson's Biological Principles. As before with the Universal Principles, we hope to have produced a clearer, more consistent and more logically integrated version of the "biological syllogism" implied in Stephenson's list. Yet again, in order to maintain the continuity of this reinterpretation with Stephenson's original work, *italics* will identify any and all edits.

No. 15. Organic Matter. (SP_{19})
The material of the body of a "living thing" is organized matter.

No. 16. Innate Intelligence. (SP_{20})
A living thing has *the intelligence of the universe inborn within it, referred to as its in*nate intelligence.

No. 17. The Chiropractic Meaning of Life. (SP_2)
The expression of this *innate* intelligence through matter is the chiropractic meaning of "life."

No. 18. The Union of Intelligence, Force and Matter (The Triune of Life). (SP_3)
Life is necessarily the union of *this* intelligence and *the* matter *of a living thing, brought about by the creation of specific internal biological forces.*

No. 19. Evidence of Life. (SP_{18})
The signs of life *(the ability to assimilate, eliminate, grow, reproduce and adapt)* are evidence of the intelligence of life.

No. 20. The Mission of Innate Intelligence. (SP_{21})
The mission of *a living thing's in*nate intelligence is to maintain the material of *its* body in active organization.

No. 21. The Perfection of the Triune. (SP$_5$)
In order to have 100% *l*ife, there must be 100% *i*ntelligence, 100% *f*orce, and 100% *m*atter.

No. 22. The Amount of Innate Intelligence. (SP$_{22}$)
There is 100% of *i*nnate *i*ntelligence in every living thing, the requisite amount, proportional to its organization.

No. 23. The Function of Innate Intelligence. (SP$_{23}$)
The function of *a living thing's i*nnate intelligence is to adapt *environmental* forces and matter for use in *its* body, so that all parts of *its* body will have coordinated action for mutual benefit.

No. 24. The Principle of Coordination. (SP$_{32}$)
Coordination is the principle of harmonious *inter*action *among* all the parts of an organism, in fulfilling their *functions* and purposes.

No. 25. The Limits of Adaptation. (SP$_{24}$)
*A living thing's i*nnate intelligence adapts forces and matter for *use in its* body as long as it can do so without breaking a universal law; *in other words, its expression* is limited by the limitations of matter *and time.*

No. 26. The Normality of Innate Intelligence. (SP$_{27}$)
*A living thing's i*nnate intelligence is always normal, and its function is always normal.

No. 27. The Character of Internal Biological Forces. (SP$_{25}$)
The forces *a living thing's i*nnate intelligence *creates are* never *intended to* injure or destroy the *living thing itself.*

No. 28. Comparison of Environmental and Internal Biological Forces. (SP$_{26}$)
In order to carry on the universal cycle of life, *environmental* forces are destructive *to a specific living thing, unless it can adapt them, whereas internal biological* forces *are* constructive *to the specific living thing that creates them, unless they suffer interference.*

No. 29. Interference with Transmission of Internal Biological Forces. (SP$_{29}$)
There can be interference with the transmission of *internal biological* forces.

No. 30. The Causes of Dis-ease. (SP$_{30}$)
Interference with the transmission of *internal biological* forces causes incoordination, *or* dis-ease.

CHAPTER 9

The "Chiropractic Principles"

Chiropractic is a philosophy, science and art of things natural; a system of adjusting the segments of the spinal column by hand only, for the correction of the cause of dis-ease.

And yet you ask, "Can Chiropractic cure appendicitis or the 'flu'?" Have you more faith in a knife or a spoonful of medicine than in the Innate power that animates the internal living world?

B. J. PALMER (1927, 1949)

To assemble the Biological Principles, we first had to sort out and set aside three of Stephenson's remaining principles, specifically SP_{28}, SP_{31} and SP_{33}, as being too specific to apply to the broad category of biological life. In light of their explicit references to the nerve system, the spinal column and vertebral subluxations, we categorized them as Chiropractic Principles. Although they form a very short list, nonetheless these three principles constitute the summative conclusion of the entire syllogism. They relate all the basic concepts explored in both the Universal Principles and the Biological Principles to the topic of primary historical focus and professional importance to chiropractors, namely the *potential* for a dysfunctional relationship between the spinal column and the nerve system, as embodied in the concept of the ***vertebral subluxation,*** to disrupt the expression of the body's innate intelligence as normal, healthy function, coordination and adaptation. These last three principles, again in Stephenson's original order and wording, are as follows:

No. 28. The Conductors of Innate Forces.
> The forces of Innate Intelligence operate through or over the nervous system in animal bodies.

No. 31. Subluxations.
> Interference with transmission in the body is always directly or indirectly due to subluxations in the spinal column.

No. 33. The Law of Demand and Supply.
> The Law of Demand and Supply is existent in the body in its ideal state; wherein the "clearing house" is the brain, Innate the virtuous "banker," brain cells "clerks," and nerve cells "messengers."

Rearranging the Chiropractic Principles:

With so few principles involved, the possibilities for rearrangement, much less the necessity of doing so, are minimal. The only rearrangement that seems logically obvious is to move SP_{33} (The Law of Demand and Supply) above SP_{31} (Subluxation). This "kills two birds with one stone." First, it places the "Law of Demand and Supply" directly after the principle identifying the primacy of the nerve system as an essential chiropractic tenet. This is perfectly reasonable, because the Law of Demand and Supply, in spite of its archaic, economic metaphorical construct, is nothing more (or less) than an elaboration of the co-ordinative and adaptive function of the nerve system introduced in SP_{28}, in terms of a metaphor of the living thing's innate intelligence as its ultimate accountant, busy balancing needs against available resources. Within the metaphor of the body as a great, vibrant community of cells, each taking from the whole what it needs for its own survival and contributing to the whole what it specializes in providing for the survival of the whole, this makes perfect sense. But it doesn't make sense as the conclusion of the entire syllogism or as a conclusion from SP_{31}. In moving it above SP_{31}, we also push SP_{31} to the very end, where it can and, in fact, *does* serve admirably as the conclusion of the entire syllogism.

STEPHENSON'S CHIROPRACTIC PRINCIPLES IN LOGICAL ORDER

We have now created a third, and final, subset of Stephenson's Principles, which are listed, as above, in their original wording but in their new order. Again, to avoid confusion and maintain the connection between Stephenson's first rough syllogism and this current work, the original order of each principle is indicated with an SP_n designation, reflecting its earlier position. As before, following this listing, these principles subsequently will be referred to by their position in the new arrangement, rather than their position in Stephenson's original list, in order to take advantage of the logical strength of our rearrangement.

No. 31. The Conductors of Innate Forces. (SP_{28})
The forces of Innate Intelligence operate through or over the nervous system in animal bodies.

No. 32. The Law of Demand and Supply. (SP_{33})
The Law of Demand and Supply is existent in the body in its ideal state; wherein the "clearing house" is the brain, Innate the virtuous "banker," brain cells "clerks," and nerve cells "messengers."

No. 33. Subluxations. (SP_{31})
Interference with transmission in the body is always directly or indirectly due to subluxations in the spinal column.

Editing the Chiropractic Principles:

Finally, we will again consider any changes in grammar or terminology that may clarify or make the chiropractic principles more logically consistent with the concepts developed in the rest of the syllogism.

Principle 31 Revised:

Principle 31 (The Conductors of Innate Forces – *The forces of Innate Intelligence operate through or over the nervous system in animal bodies.*), like the closely related Principle 33 (Subluxations – *Interference with transmission in the body is **always** directly or indirectly due to subluxations in the spinal column.*), suffers from an unsupportable exclusivity of concept. It correctly addresses the topic of interest in the traditional chiropractic clinical paradigm, namely the coordinating and adapting forces being created and transmitted by the functioning neurons in living organisms with nerve systems (which Stephenson's identifies as *animal bodies),* but its wording clearly implies that these are *"The* forces of Innate Intelligence" as if they were the only forces that can be attributed to the functioning of a living thing's innate intelligence.

But Stephenson's earlier principles evolve the concept that *all of the internal biological forces* being created within the physiological workings of a living organism are created by the intelligence indigenous to and responsible for its overall organization. If this is the case, then unless the forces being created and transmitted over the nerve system are the *only internal biological forces being created* within animal bodies, which is clearly not the case, there are other "forces of Innate Intelligence" to which this principle does not refer. Indeed, hormonal forces, muscular forces, skeletal biomechanical forces, even the chemical forces of energy transfer (the Krebs Cycle, *ATP/ADP,* etc.) are *all* internal biological forces, in which case the forces operating through or over the nerve system in vertebrates are, in fact, only *some of the forces* being created by a living thing's innate intelligence. Accordingly, this principle needs to be reworded to reflect this fact, and to make it congruent with the argument we elaborated in revising Principle 27 (see above). This is easily accomplished by simply saying "In animal bodies,[25] **some of** the forces a living thing's innate intelligence creates operate through or over its nerve system."[26]

Principle 32 Revised:

Principle 32 (The Law of Demand and Supply – *The Law of Demand and Supply is existent in the body in its ideal state; wherein the "clearing house" is the*

---

[25]Note that the phrase *in animal bodies* is moved to the front of the principle, but not altered.
[26]Note also the use of *nerve system,* instead of *nervous system.*

brain, Innate the virtuous "banker," brain cells "clerks," and nerve cells "messengers.") seems to stand out as an archaic and metaphorical anachronism in Stephenson's list of principles. However, if we look at it *in this position* in the syllogism, following directly upon the introduction of the topic of the function of the nerve system as a conductor of some of the forces a living thing's innate intelligence creates, its role in the argument is very clear, even if Stephenson's choice of metaphor is outdated. It is simply here to correctly attribute the significance of the forces being transmitted over the nerve system, to the overall organization of the multi-cellular body as conceived by the living thing's innate intelligence and expressed through the coordination of all the needs and resources (the "balancing of accounts" implied by Stephenson's banking metaphor) of all the individual constituents (the tissue cells) of the body's collective community.

> **This principle then stands not as an economic metaphor for, but as a simple physiological model of, the *primacy of the nerve system.***

Once this is understood, it is a simple matter to update and "de-metaphorize" this principle, by stating it in basic neurological terms congruent with our current understanding of the overall coordinating function of the nerve system in the body's biological economy. To achieve this, a total rewrite of the same concept is proposed along these lines: *"The Law of Demand and Supply operates and is expressed in animal bodies through the functioning of the nerve system; wherein the brain acts as a CPU (Central Processing Unit) for the living thing's innate intelligence, and wherein the nerves transmit messages from the body to the brain, concerning its needs (demands), and transmit messages from the brain to the body to meet (supply) those needs."* This principle then stands not as an economic metaphor for, but as a simple physiological model of, the *primacy of the nerve system* in managing the challenges of the cellular specialization and mutual interdependence of the vast community of cells that constitute a neurologically coordinated multi-cellular organism.

Principle 33 Revised:

Principle 33 (Subluxations – *Interference with transmission in the body is always directly or indirectly due to subluxations in the spinal column.*), like Principle 31 (in its original form), has been a source of heated argument over its logically unsupportable absolutism, in this case centered on the single word "always." The absolutism implied by this one word is problematic on several levels. In terms of "always," must this principle, like Principle 31, be interpreted to imply that nerve forces are the only internal biological forces being created by a living thing's innate intelligence? If not, as we argued above, then it seems logically inconsistent to conclude that, of all the forces being created at all levels of the body's functioning, only "nerve forces" are vulnerable to interference. According to Principle 12, *"There can be interference with the transmission of universal forces."* According to Principle 28, *"There can be interference with the transmission of internal biological forces."* Must there be neurological interference before it is even possible for a blood clot to *interfere with the transmission of* hemoglobin-bound oxygen (an internal biological force, created by a living thing's innate intelligence and necessary for function and survival, if ever there was one) to the heart muscle or brain? The forces being transmitted over the nerve system are *only some of the forces* a living thing's innate intelligence utilizes to create function, coordination, adaptation and health. The concept of interference must logically apply to the other forces also. Thus we must insert our first qualification into Stephenson's original principle: *"Interference with **the**[27] transmission of **nerve forces** in the body is always directly or indirectly due to subluxations in the spinal column."*

In terms of "always," must this principle be interpreted to imply that all organisms that "create nerve impulses" have spinal columns? The taxonomy of currently living species tells us that this is not so. We know of many forms of life that have nerve systems but do not form their skeletal frame around a central spinal column. Clearly, the interference to which this principle is referring is related to the specific biomechanical and physiological consequences of the intimate relationship that exists between the spinal cord and the bony articulations of the spinal column that is unique to the *vertebrata*. Thus we must insert our second qualification into Stephenson's original principle: *"**In vertebrates**, interference with the transmission of nerve forces in the body is always directly or indirectly due to subluxations in the spinal column."*

Lastly, must this principle be interpreted to imply that, even in terms of the nerve forces being transmitted over the nerve systems through the spinal columns of vertebrates, only the relatively mild articular trauma referred to as "subluxation" can create interference? Surely there must be other forms of interference to which they are susceptible, in addition to those directly, or even indirectly attributable to the spinal column's potential to misalign slightly. To postulate that nerve impulses are only vulnerable to interference via subluxation is to contradict the obvious vulnerability of nerve tissue to the other kinds of trauma as well. Must there be a subluxation in the moment before a bullet can penetrate, shatter the spinal column and rupture the spinal cord directly? This is an argument *ad absurdum* to defend the indefensible – that **all** interference "is directly or indirectly due to subluxations in the spinal column."

This may lead us to wonder what argument drove the need for the insertion of this "exclusive qualifier" on the concept of interference to innate forces in the

---

[27] Note that the insertion of "the" before "transmission" is purely grammatical.

first place. Why does a syllogism that posits a model of interference as the fundamental obstacle to the perfect expression of the intelligence of the entire universe come down to the concept that the only possible source of interference in the entire human being is subluxation of the spinal column? Perhaps we might conclude that the "always" in this final principle is more of a political statement of the need for the chiropractic profession to elevate and ennoble its chosen clinical focus on the vertebral subluxation with philosophic and ideological significance over and above that which is purely logically defensible. In any event, to bring our final principle into congruence with the entire model created by the syllogism we have been working so hard to strengthen, this argument will be much better served if we replace the absolute term "always" with the more easily defensible concept that *"In vertebrates, interference with the transmission of nerve forces in the body is **often** directly or indirectly due to subluxations in the spinal column."*

STEPHENSON'S CHIROPRACTIC PRINCIPLES REARRANGED AND EDITED

With the completion of the thirty-third of Stephenson's Principles, we have completed our initial work on Stephenson's Chiropractic Principles, and on the syllogism as a whole. As before, with both the Universal and the Biological Principles, we hope to have produced a clearer, more consistent and more logically integrated version of this portion of the syllogism. Again, in order to maintain the continuity of this reinterpretation with Stephenson's original work, changes from Stephenson's original formulations of these principles are identified by *italics*.

No. 31. **The Conductors of Internal Biological Forces. (SP$_{28}$)**
   In animal bodies, *some of* the forces *a living thing's i*nnate intelligence *creates* operate through or over the nerve system.

No. 32. **The Law of Demand and Supply. (SP$_{33}$)**
   The Law of Demand and Supply *operates and is expressed in animal bodies through the functioning of the nerve system; wherein the brain acts as a CPU (Central Processing Unit) for the living thing's innate intelligence, and wherein the nerves transmit messages from the body to the brain, concerning its needs (demands), and transmit messages from the brain to the body to meet (supply) those needs.*

No. 33. **Subluxations. (SP$_{31}$)**
   In vertebrates, interference with *the* transmission *of nerve forces* in the body is *often* directly or indirectly due to subluxations in the spinal column.

CHAPTER 10

Conclusions

Our efforts will have been rewarded by the creation of a better, clearer model of the concept of an intelligent universe continuously organizing matter into myriad complex structures, including living human beings, through the use of forces that carry intelligence's intent to matter to be expressed as its organization, and, in living organisms, as function and health.

We have arrived at the culmination of our initial efforts to rearrange and edit Stephenson's Principles into a stronger, clearer, more logical argument. As with any deductive syllogism, ultimately it will need to be judged by how well it creates a model of reality that we can understand and, more importantly, apply in useful ways. Let's take one final look at the "finished product" and see if it reads more smoothly, clearly and connectedly. If it does, our efforts will have been rewarded by the creation of a better, clearer model of the concept of an intelligent universe continuously organizing itself into myriad complex structures, including living human beings, through the use of forces that carry intelligence's intent to matter to be expressed as its organization, and, in living organisms, as function and health.

THE UNIVERSAL PRINCIPLES:

No. 1. The Major Premise.
> There is a universal intelligence in all matter, continuously giving to it all its properties and actions, thus maintaining it in existence, and giving this intelligence its expression.

No. 2. Cause and Effect.
> Every effect has causes and every cause has effects.

No. 3. The Principle of Time.
> All processes require time.

No. 4. No Organization without the Effort of Force.
> Matter can have no organization without the application of force by intelligence.

No. 5. Universal Expression.
Force is manifested as organization in matter; all matter has organization, therefore there is universal intelligence expressed in all matter.

No. 6. The Triune of Organization.
Any organized structure is a triunity having three necessary factors; namely, intelligence, matter and the force which unites them.

No. 7. The Function of Intelligence.
The function of intelligence is to create force.

No. 8. The Amount of Intelligence in Matter.
The amount of intelligence for any given amount of matter is 100%, and is always proportional to its requirements.

No. 9. The Function of Force.
The function of force is to unite intelligence and matter.

No. 10. The Amount of Force Created by Intelligence.
The amount of force created by intelligence is always 100%.

No. 11. The Character of Universal Forces.
The forces the universe's intelligence creates throughout the universe are manifested as physical laws; are unswerving and unadapted, and have no solitude for the structures in which they work.

No. 12. Interference with the Transmission of Universal Forces.
There can be interference with the transmission of universal forces.

No. 13. The Function of Matter.
The function of matter is to express force.

No. 14. Intelligence in Both Organic and Inorganic Matter.
Universal intelligence gives force to both organic and inorganic matter.

THE BIOLOGICAL PRINCIPLES

No. 15. Organic Matter.
The material of the body of a "living thing" is organized matter.

No. 16. Innate Intelligence.
A living thing has the intelligence of the universe inborn within it, referred to as its innate intelligence.

No. 17. The Chiropractic Meaning of Life.
The expression of this innate intelligence through matter is the chiropractic meaning of "life."

No. 18. The Union of Intelligence, Force and Matter (The Triune of Life).
Life is necessarily the union of this intelligence and the matter of a living thing, brought about by the creation of specific internal biological forces.

No. 19. Evidence of Life.
The signs of life (the ability to assimilate, eliminate, grow, reproduce and adapt) are evidence of the intelligence of life.

No. 20. The Mission of Innate Intelligence.
The mission of a living thing's innate intelligence is to maintain the material of its body in active organization.

No. 21. The Perfection of the Triune.
In order to have 100% life, there must be 100% intelligence, 100% force, and 100% matter.

No. 22. The Amount of Innate Intelligence.
There is 100% of innate intelligence in every living thing, the requisite amount, proportional to its organization.

No. 23. The Function of Innate Intelligence.
The function of a living thing's innate intelligence is to adapt environmental forces and matter for use in its body, so that all parts of its body will have coordinated action for mutual benefit.

No. 24. The Principle of Coordination.
Coordination is the principle of harmonious interaction among all the parts of an organism, in fulfilling their functions and purposes.

No. 25. The Limits of Adaptation.
A living thing's innate intelligence adapts forces and matter for use in its body as long as it can do so without breaking a universal law; in other words, its expression is limited by the limitations of matter and time.

No. 26. The Normality of Innate Intelligence.
A living thing's innate intelligence is always normal, and its function is always normal.

No. 27. **The Character of Internal Biological Forces.**
The forces a living thing's innate intelligence creates are never intended to injure or destroy the living thing itself.

No. 28. **Comparison of Environmental and Internal Biological Forces.**
In order to carry on the universal cycle of life, environmental forces are destructive to a specific living thing, unless it can adapt them, whereas internal biological forces are constructive to the specific living thing that creates them, unless they suffer interference.

No. 29. **Interference with Transmission of Internal Biological Forces.**
There can be interference with the transmission of internal biological forces.

No. 30. **The Causes of Dis-ease.**
Interference with the transmission of internal biological forces causes incoordination, or dis-ease.

THE CHIROPRACTIC PRINCIPLES

No. 31. **The Conductors of Internal Biological Forces.**
In animals, some of the forces a living thing's innate intelligence creates operate through or over its nerve system.

No. 32. **The Law of Demand and Supply.**
The Law of Demand and Supply operates and is expressed in animal bodies through the functioning of the nerve system; wherein the brain acts as a CPU (Central Processing Unit) for the living thing's innate intelligence, and wherein the nerves transmit messages from the body to the brain, concerning its needs (demands), and transmit messages from the brain to the body to meet (supply) those needs.

No. 33. **Subluxations.**
In vertebrates, interference with the transmission of nerve forces in the body is often directly or indirectly due to subluxations in the spinal column.

The Wider Applicability of "Chiropractic's" Principles:
With this substantial reorganization and reevaluation of the language and sequencing of these principles, one conclusion that emerges is that chiropractic's basic metaphysical concepts (universal intelligence, innate intelligence, force,

interference) are not exclusively applicable to chiropractic, either as a clinical practice or as a profession. In fact, it is only in the last three principles, and specifically in the exploration of the implications of the last clause of the last principle in the entire syllogism[28] that the entire "science and art" of chiropractic, focused around the value of the primary chiropractic intervention, i.e. the specific chiropractic adjustment, have their origins.

To illustrate this, if we were to replace our last three principles, the specifically "Chiropractic Principles," with other principles that might be considered equally consistent with the first thirty principles, we could theoretically formulate the basis for the clinical science, art and profession known as *acupuncture.* Thus we might find ourselves "sharing a philosophy" with another profession, based on the recognition of the centrality of the body's innate intelligence in health and function, but not necessarily focused on the relationship between the nerve system, the spinal column and healthy function. Consider the following three ***hypothetical*** principles, which I just made up "off the top of my head:"

No. 31. The Transmission of the Internal Biological Force called "Chi."
In human beings, some of the forces a person's innate intelligence creates operate through or over non-anatomically defined channels called "meridians." Such internal, biological forces are referred to as "chi."

No. 32. The Law of Yin/Yang Balance.
The Law of Yin/Yang Balance operates and is expressed in animal bodies through the flow of *chi* through the body's meridians; wherein the innate intelligence of the body uses the unobstructed and balanced flow of *chi* (positive and negative *yin/yang*) to maintain harmonic balance among the body's own constituent parts and to maintain the body in harmony with any positive and negative environmental influences that may affect it.

No. 33. Chi Imbalances.
In human beings, interference with the flow of chi in the body is often directly or indirectly due to obstructions to and/or imbalances between or among the several meridians of the body.

Theoretically, these three principles, substituted for the Chiropractic Principles, could just as well complete this syllogism as the underlying metaphysical basis for acupuncture. Thus, acupuncture, like chiropractic, could also be founded on the same principles (the Universal and Biological Principles above) that

---

[28] "In vertebrates, interference with the transmission of nerve forces in the body is ***often directly or indirectly due to subluxations in the spinal column.***"

recognize and define the role of a universal intelligence in the organization of matter, its role in living things as the body's innate intelligence, the role of the creation, transmission and expression of forces in the connection between the organizing intent of intelligence and the manifestation of that intent in matter, and the unobstructed functioning of this linkage as the fundamental basis of health and vitality.

Of course, we must also recognize that this does not make acupuncture and chiropractic the same thing. Indeed, what this best illustrates is that whether you choose to practice chiropractic or acupuncture does not necessarily depend on whether you recognize the innate intelligence of life, but on whether you consider vertebral subluxations or *chi* imbalances as the most important *interference to the expression of the body's innate intelligence*. In the end, if we set aside questions of differing professional definitions and competing scopes of practice, we might actually ask ourselves, "What health care profession *wouldn't want* to base itself on these very principles of the existence of a universal intelligence, the *innate intelligence* of life, the forces intelligence continuously creates, which are expressed by matter as organization and health, and the devastating consequences of *interference* to the communication between intelligence and matter that underlies the very nature of existence itself?"

PART TWO

Chiropractic's "Normal Complete Cycle"

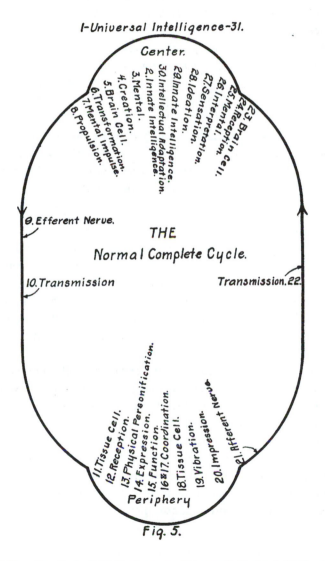

The Normal Complete Cycle, R.W. Stephenson, *Chiropractic Textbook*, 1948, p. 11

CHAPTER 11

Introduction

The Normal Complete Cycle is the outline of the story of the normal functioning of Innate in the body. In this cycle thirty-one steps are named. There are sixteen in the efferent half and fifteen in the afferent half. All the steps of the cycle are the names of units of force, processes, matter, and places. As the C. G. S.[29] system is the fundamental unit system in the study of physics and mathematics, so the forun, mental impulse, and tissue cell are fundamental units in Chiropractic.

R. W. STEPHENSON (1927)

The second section of this work will review the Normal Complete Cycle,[30] which is Stephenson's model of the relationship between awareness and response that underlies the neurological control of all living functions and adaptations. This model is an expansion of the concepts embodied in Principle 32 (above).

No. 32. The Law of Demand and Supply

The Law of Demand and Supply operates and is expressed in animal bodies through the functioning of the nerve system; wherein the brain acts as a CPU (central processing unit) for the living thing's innate intelligence, and wherein the nerves transmit messages from the body to the brain, concerning its needs (demands), and transmit messages from the brain to the body to meet (supply) those needs.

The Normal Complete Cycle forms the second great philosophical challenge in understanding Stephenson's (and B. J. Palmer's) grand metaphysical vision. If we think of Stephenson's Thirty-Three Principles as the dry, academic, logical arguments that underlie and support the concept of the fundamental *intelligence* of the universe, its tendency toward *self-organization*, and its most dramatic and amazing expression as the phenomenon of *life*, then the Normal Complete Cycle is the hustle and bustle, the dynamic rhythms and pulses, the very ebb and flow of the living expression of that intelligence in the adaptive and coordinative actions, reactions, reflexes and responses mediated by the forces created, trans-

---

[29] *(C)entimeter, (G)ram, (S)econd – three basic units of measurement in physics*
[30] Stephenson's *Chiropractic Textbook*, 1948 ed., Articles 49–101, pp. 17–65

mitted and expressed "through or over [the] nerve system" in those forms of life that have one.

If there is an *innate intelligence* acting in living things, where and how does it touch the body itself? How can it *(intelligence)* change *matter's* actions? How does it "know" what the body's "needs" are? How does what happens in its environment impact and *change* where, when and how a living thing must act, react and respond to maintain, sustain and recreate itself, moment by moment? This is where the rubber meets the road; where the ideality of our metaphysics collides with the reality of a vast number of mostly cohesive, all genetically identical yet surprisingly dif-

> If there is an *innate intelligence* acting in living things, where and how does it touch the body itself?

ferentiated, highly specialized, sticky, wiggly, infinitesimal cells conglomerated into a single, self-assembling, self-maintaining, self-repairing and self-evolving *being* called *you.* This is where the effervescent idea of an immaterial *intelligence* meets the everyday concreteness of the living processes of the physical body. The Normal Complete Cycle is our attempt to capture, with intellectual "stop-action photography," the interactive, communicative dynamism of this self-sustaining whirlwind of interrelatedness, this *symphony of function,* as it is created by and unfolds through the relationship between the body's *consciousness of itself and its environment* and the forces that drive, coordinate and adapt its immensely complex panoply of internal physiological activities and external physical actions.

Perhaps no other example could better illustrate the sheer, overwhelming physicality of this process we are about to consider than the concept of the actual physical time frame we will be considering as we examine just one single iteration of the Normal Complete Cycle. Consider the speed with which the neurological communication of a signal to alter and/or adjust any given physiological response can be sent. From its summative creation in the cortex of the brain to its reception and expression as a change in muscle tonus in your big toe, a simple motor impulse can "make the trip" in just about 5 *milliseconds.* This leads us to realize that the body's *innate intelligence,* creating adaptive motor impulses as quickly and as often as needed, can "adjust" the precise tonus of the muscles of your big toe somewhere around *two hundred times per second.* In other words, after you finish studying how the Normal Complete Cycle describes the continual and ongoing relationship between the body's *intelligence* and its physiology, step back and ponder the significance of the fact that this actual, partially physical relationship can change the body's actions twelve thousand times every minute over each and every nerve fiber in your entire body.

Unfortunately, the neurophysiologists and the psychologists pigeon-hole all of this and dismiss the nearly overwhelming and humbling significance of such a biologically vast intelligence by labeling it the *sub-conscious mind,* or the *unconscious mind* or (my favorite) the *autonomic nerve system.* If we learn one thing from our exploration of the Normal Complete Cycle, it is that the body's innate intelligence is neither sub-conscious nor unconscious; rather it is the body's total *hyper-consciousness* of itself and everything that happens within it and/or to the matter of which it is composed. It is actually the "higher" cortical functions of my brain, which I think of as my "self-consciousness," that is almost completely unconscious of everything that is going on inside me (and is usually not really *that aware* of what is going on all around me, most of the time). Thus, it is with a certain sense of humility, and not without a certain sense of irony, that we will look at the Normal Complete Cycle, and ponder the idea that the *intelligence* of the entire universe, embodied in the self-created organization of our own few pounds of its matter, expresses itself as fully and completely as it can in each and every nerve impulse we create and in response to each and every internal and external environmental change, variation and challenge we are faced with.

> If we learn one thing from our exploration of the Normal Complete Cycle, it is that the body's innate intelligence is neither sub-conscious nor unconscious; rather it is the body's *hyper-consciousness* of itself and everything that happens within it.

As presented in Stephenson's *Chiropractic Textbook,* the Normal Complete Cycle is an expansion and a sophistication of the Simple Cycle.[31] The Simple Cycle defines, in the simplest possible terms, the relationship between innate intelligence and the matter (tissue cells, organs and glands) of a living organism with a nerve system. The Normal Complete Cycle, on the other hand, expands on the concepts of the six simple steps of the Simple Cycle *(Creation, Efferent Transmission, Expression, Impression, Afferent Transmission and Interpretation),* looking at each step more closely and analyzing each step into its conceptual components.

It follows the same basic format as the Simple Cycle, tracing the flow of efferent information from its conception by intelligence, through transmission via force, to its expression as a specific change in matter's motion (and hence a change in the adaptive actions of the living organism.) From that point, the Normal Complete Cycle then traces the flow of afferent information back from the momentary state of the matter's motion, through transmission via impression, to its reception and analysis by intelligence in the mental realm.

---

[31]*Ibid.* Art. 36, p. 7

Like the Simple Cycle, the Normal Complete Cycle is formatted in "steps." These steps represent the sequential nature of the cyclical process.[32] In the Simple Cycle, each step is the action consequent to the previous step. However the "steps" in the Normal Complete Cycle extend beyond this, and may represent actors (what is doing the action), or locations (in what realm, at what location or in what tissue the action is occurring), as well as the actions themselves. This is the primary way in which the Normal Complete Cycle expands upon the simplicity of the Simple Cycle.

To understand the Normal Complete Cycle, the reader must recall and review some basic concepts of chiropractic philosophy derived from the Thirty-Three Principles and the Triune of Organization/Life. Let us begin with some germane definitions. These definitions are *paraphrased* from the concepts developed in R. W. Stephenson's *Chiropractic Textbook*.

Basic Philosophic Definitions:

Universal intelligence:[33] The necessary assumed cause of all organization

Innate intelligence:[34] Universal intelligence being expressed in a living organism

Mental realm:[35] The immaterial (non-physical) aspect of reality which is the location of the activities of universal/innate intelligence

Physical (material) realm:[36] Matter and energy located in and moving through time and space

Innate brain:[37] The organ used by the body's innate intelligence to assemble mental impulses

Innate mind:[38] The innate brain actively expressing the body's innate intelligence

Innate body:[39] Those tissue cells that receive mental impulses from the innate mind to direct and coordinate their function

Point of creation: The physical site where intelligence introduces new informational content (a new message) into an energetic transformation, thereby creating a distinct, new force

---

[32] *Ibid.* Art. 37, p. 8
[33] *Ibid.* Art. 49, p. 17
[34] *Ibid.* Art. 50, p. 17
[35] *Ibid.* Art. 52, p. 21
[36] *Ibid.* Art. 58, p. 26
[37] *Ibid.* Art. 43, p. 13
[38] *Ibid.* Art. 54, p. 23
[39] *Ibid.* Art. 45, p. 14

Transmission:[40] The movement of a force from the point of its creation to the point of its intended expression

Point of intended expression: The material structure the motions or actions of which intelligence designs a specific force to change or influence

Mental impulse:[41] An efferent nerve impulse created by the innate mind to carry adaptive information to a specific tissue cell of the innate body

The Nature of Cycles:

In studying the Normal Complete Cycle, it is important to remember that, as with any cycle, the starting point of the Normal Complete Cycle is arbitrary. A cycle is a repeated series of similar events which tends to return to *any point* in the cycle. Thus a cycle can be said to *start at any point* in the series.

However, in chiropractic philosophy, it has been traditional to start the description of cycles of adaptation at the point where intelligence *(innate intelligence* in this case, since intelligence is acting through the matter of a particular living thing) *initiates an organizational change* in matter's motion. Since the Normal Complete Cycle is a description of a living thing with a nerve system, it is appropriate to identify the starting point with the creation of the *efferent nerve impulse* or "mental impulse." The first steps of the Normal Complete Cycle are therefore called the **efferent side of the cycle.** At the same time, it is crucial to note that, in this use of the term "efferent," we are not referring just to the flow of influence from brain to body, as the neuro-physiologist might. We are referring to the flow of information from the *innate intelligence* of the body to the physical matter of the body. The concept that the physical efferent side of the cycle starts from the brain is the result of the concept that innate intelligence uses the brain to assemble, and the nerve system to transmit, the specific forces that carry this flow of information. It actually starts first with universal intelligence![42]

At the point at which intelligence has successfully altered the motions/ actions of matter, the Normal Complete Cycle begins to describe the return of information from the physical realm back to the mental realm, to allow intelligence's awareness of matter's organization to form. From this point forward, the steps of the Normal Complete Cycle will be referred to as the **afferent side of the cycle.**[43] Of course, it is crucial to remember in this discussion that the Normal Complete Cycle is a cycle. As in any cycle, the afferent steps will ultimately lead back to the efferent side of the cycle, and the cycle will repeat itself.

---

[40] *Ibid.* Art. 62, p. 31
[41] *Ibid.* Art. 59, p. 29
[42] *Ibid.* Art. 50, p. 17
[43] *Ibid.* Art. 86, p. 52

CHAPTER 12

The Efferent Side of the Normal Complete Cycle

In an orchestra, the thought of an integrated symphony of sound is communicated from the mind of the conductor to the minds of the musicians by the smallest and least significant piece of orchestral equipment, the lowly baton. Yet, it is this connection that creates the mind of the orchestra itself, and thus creates the symphony, which is the expression of that "orchestral mind."

STEP 1: Universal Intelligence[44]

The first step of the Normal Complete Cycle is *Universal Intelligence,* an "actor" in the process we are describing. This is a suitable starting point in describing the organization and responses of a living organism, simply because *all* organization is caused by the universe's ability to organize itself. On the other hand, we would certainly wish to denote that this universal cause of organization is, more specifically, operating through the specific matter of a specific living organism.[45] This leads directly to the second step of the Normal Complete Cycle.

Universal Intelligence is a suitable starting point in describing the organization and responses of a living organism, simply because all organization is caused by the universe's ability to organize itself.

STEP 2: Innate Intelligence[46]

The second step of the Normal Complete Cycle is *Innate Intelligence.* This denotes that the cycle of adaptation in a specific living organism starts and ends with the organizing intelligence of the universe operating within and through the substance (the matter and energy) of that living organism. Thus we refer to the organizing intelligence of the universe as the inborn organizing intelligence of that specific living organism, in other words, its *innate intelligence.*

Innate Intelligence further denotes that the activities of this organizing intelligence are devoted to *maintaining the organization* of that particular, specific living organism. This is actually an expression of a universal principle. When working within a molecule, the forces that the universe's intelligence creates

---

[44] *Ibid.* Art. 49, p. 17
[45] Principle 16 – A living thing has the intelligence of the universe inborn within it, referred to as its innate intelligence, p. 78 above
[46] Stephenson's *Chiropractic Textbook,* 1948 ed., Art. 50, p. 17

internally (within the molecule itself) are constructive to the organization of that molecule, whereas a force created by universal intelligence outside of a molecule would not necessarily be created to be constructive to that molecule. If such a force were to impinge on that particular molecule, it would tend to disorganize that molecule.

This principle is even more clearly evident when intelligence is operating within and outside of a living organism. Intelligence operating outside of a living organism (universal intelligence) will create forces (environmental forces) that are not necessarily designed to re-establish, maintain or enhance the specific organization of that living organism.[47] On the other hand, that same organizing intelligence, when operating within a specific living organism (its *innate intelligence),* will be creating forces (internal biological forces) that *are* specifically intended to be constructive to the organization of that specific living organism. Thus *innate intelligence* denotes the constructive quality of the activity of intelligence *relative to the needs of the particular, specific living organism* being considered.[48]

Finally, innate intelligence is the immaterial actor in *adaptation.* This intelligence, the infinite organizational creativity of the universe itself, will function continuously to accomplish its mission of creating and maintaining the organization of the living organism. That function will be to create the specific information that will form the specific responses (changes in matter's motion) that will maintain the living organism's optimum organization (health) in the face of any and all challenges to that organization.

STEP 3: Mental Realm[49]

The third step of the Normal Complete Cycle is titled *Mental Realm.* This "step" denotes the *location* of the activity of intelligence. Even though we understand that *intelligence,* being an *immaterial* organizational causality, has *no physical location,* it is conceptually convenient to assign a name to the "immaterial location" of intelligence's existence and therefore its activity.

It is philosophically crucial, however, to avoid the conceptual trap of thinking of the mental realm as being located within the head or brain of an organism. Indeed, the mental realm applies to the activity of intelligence in creating organization from the atomic to the galactic physical scale. In any and all cases, the mental realm refers to the "immaterial dimension" or "immaterial aspect" of reality, and not a location within the physical universe. If we wish to try to conceptualize it, a useful metaphor may be that the mental realm is another "dimension" that touches the physical realm *at every point* of its existence. To get

---

[47]*Ibid.* Art. 327, p. 251
[48]*Ibid.* Art. 342, p. 263
[49]*Ibid.* Art. 52, p. 21

from the physical to the mental realm, we do not need to "go" anywhere. We only need to cross a *material/immaterial* boundary, or *interface*. The "activities" that occur in the mental realm are the activities of intelligence, including its awareness of the organization of matter, its judgment of the "needs" of specific organized structures and its creation of the information necessary to maintain or alter the organization of specific organized structures.

STEP 4: Creation[50]

The fourth step of the Normal Complete Cycle is *Creation*. This step represents the first action described in the Normal Complete Cycle. It is also significant that this is the ***first step*** of the Stephenson's simplified version of the Norman Complete Cycle, the Simple Cycle.[51] In an interesting side note, Stephenson's Simple Cycle is often referred to as the "Safety Pin Cycle," for no other reason than that the illustration of it in Stephenson's *Chiropractic Textbook* looks somewhat like a safety pin.[52] According to Stephenson, the Simple Cycle consists of three *efferent steps (Creation, Transmission* and *Expression)* followed by three *afferent steps (Impression, Transmission* and *Interpretation).* I will note each of the subsequent steps in the Simple Cycle as we come upon them, embedded within the Normal Complete Cycle.

Creation refers to the creation of specific 'bits' of information, which are the adaptive messages that the body's innate intelligence deems necessary to send to specific tissue cells to maintain or alter their physical, metabolic and/or functional activities. Each of these bits of adaptive information, which innate intelligence intends to be expressed as a specific adaptive response of a specific tissue cell or group of tissue cells, is called a ***forun.*** Stephenson puts it this way, "When Innate assembles universal forces in the brain cell they are in the form of thoughts. In this non-specific state they are called foruns. They are, as yet, thought; absolutely abstract, but the most powerful creations in nature, notwithstanding."[53]

The term *"forun"* is a word early chiropractic philosophers coined to fill a need. As we can well imagine, in 1927 there was no common term for the 'immaterial informational content of a single unitary message from intelligence to matter.' In this sense, forun will do as well as any other term. A forun, then, exist first as a thought by the living organism's innate intelligence as to what specific organizational change is necessary to adapt that living organism to the

---

[50] *Ibid.* Art. 56, p. 24
[51] *Ibid.* Art. 36, p. 7
[52] I quit using this familiar name for it in the classroom when it dawned on me that, with the advent of Velcro® fastened baby diapers, many of my students had never seen, much less used, an actual safety pin.
[53] Stephenson's *Chiropractic Textbook,* 1948 ed., Art. 58, p. 28

immediate adaptive challenges facing it.

It must be noted that the foruns created in this step of the Normal Complete Cycle must be the result of awareness on the part of the body's innate intelligence as to what has happened to that living organism in its immediate past and what its current state of organization is. Such an innate awareness presupposes an afferent process through which the body's innate intelligence forms the awareness necessary to create the appropriate information needed to meet its current adaptive challenges.

This afferent process (of the body's innate intelligence generating a perfect awareness of the body's current organization and challenges) is the subject of the second half of the Normal Complete Cycle. In starting with the efferent side, we are assuming that the afferent process has already occurred in at least one, and usually in uncounted prior manifestations of the Normal Complete Cycle. Thus, the foruns created in this step of this particular adaptive cycle are the result of the innate awareness of the body's needs created in the previous adaptive cycle.

The body's innate intelligence must, can and will create as many foruns in any one iteration of the Normal Complete Cycle as are necessary to alter matter's motion so that the organism can survive and express its potentials. In a practical sense, and considering the role of the central nerve system as the primary communications network, this means one forun per efferent nerve impulse created. Since the brain creates billions of nerve impulses per second, we would have to infer that the body's innate intelligence correspondingly creates billions of foruns per second, one message per efferent nerve impulse. Thus, each forun represents the innate thought that goes into one nerve message.

STEP 5: Brain Cell[54]

The fifth step of the Normal Complete Cycle is named *Brain Cell.* This step represents both a location and an actor in the process of adaptation. It is a *location* in that it is the site of what must happen next for an adaptation to occur, namely, the assembly of a specific *internal biological force* within the physical realm. Since "force" implies the insertion of information (in this case, the forun) into a specific type of energy (in this case, an efferent nerve impulse), the next action has to occur somewhere in the physical realm. *Brain cell* identifies where the physical aspect of this process occurs.

The "actor" to which this step refers is a specific cell of the *innate brain,*[55] the organ used by the body's innate intelligence to assemble mental impulses. This designation (innate brain) is a purely physiological designation. Anatomically, innate brain (and therefore the brain cell denoted in this step of the Normal Com-

[54] *Ibid.* Art. 57, p. 25
[55] *Ibid.* Art. 43, p. 13

plete Cycle) refers to any neuron in the central nerve system that is capable of initiating an efferent action potential along its cell membrane. The designation of the brain/spinal cord structure as *innate brain* simply identifies this physiological role of this tissue.

The brain's function as *innate brain* stands in contrast to its function as *educated brain,*[56] referring to this same tissue's other important capability. Distinct from its role in creating mental impulses, the brain also serves as the substrate for the organism's ability to accumulate, store, process and respond to specific information gathered physically from the surrounding environment and/or the organism's own internal environment. However, these computational and analytical abilities of the brain are learned responses of this tissue, whereas its function as *innate brain* in assembling mental impulses is inherent in the structure of nerve tissue itself. Thus the designation *innate brain* implies its *inborn* function, as opposed to its learned *(educated)* functions.

In the Normal Complete Cycle, *brain cell* also denotes the next actor in the process. As an actor, the brain cell has a vital role to play. It is the transformer that takes energy in one form and changes it into energy in another form. Like an electrical generator that takes the energy of falling water, burning coal or nuclear fission and transforms it into electricity, the brain cell creates the nerve impulse out of the body's store of precursor energy (perhaps best represented by the ATP molecule produced by the combustion of sugar).

With the physical transformation of one form of energy into another, a specific new force is created. The physical properties of this force are derived from the physical mechanisms of the transformer, the neuron. On the other hand, the immaterial information inserted into the force at the point of its creation must be the forun, that specific adaptive message the mental impulse is being assembled to carry. The nerve impulse, as a specific form of energy, is created by the physiology of the brain cell. The forun, as a specific bit of information, is created by the body's innate intelligence.

STEP 6: Transformation[57] (a.k.a. Efferent Transformation)[58]

The sixth step of the Normal Complete Cycle is *Transformation.*[59] This step is one of the two most difficult steps to discuss. *Transformation* and *Afferent Transmission* (renamed *"Efferent Transformation"* and *"Afferent Transformation"* in Step 22 below) both represent the actual interface between the immaterial and the

---

[56] *Ibid.* Art. 44, p. 13
[57] *Ibid.* Art. 58, p. 26
[58] See Step 22 below
[59] Stephenson's *Chiropractic Textbook,* 1948 ed., Art. 58, p. 26: "Transformation: Changing force from the mental realm to the material realm. Making a force out of a thought so that it can be physical enough to 'get a grip' on matter."

physical realms. *Efferent Transformation* denotes the "movement" of immaterial information from the purely mental realm, where it is created by the body's innate intelligence, into the physical realm, where it can be carried within a force.

What is transformed is the forun. In the mental realm, a forun is merely innate intelligence's "thought" of a specific adaptive message it needs to send to a specific tissue cell. When an actual mental impulse is assembled in the *innate brain,* this innate thought becomes changed into the specific informational content of a physical force. The forun is transformed from (potential) information "floating around" in the mental realm, into actual information (potential *form*) traveling through the physical realm. This transformation occurs in the *innate brain* as this organ expresses the body's innate intelligence through its functioning. The activity of the *innate brain* expressing the body's innate intelligence, and thereby assembling mental impulses out of foruns and nerve impulses, is called *innate mind.*[60] This is the *point of creation* of this particular type of internal biological force.

> **"Transformation" represents the *actual interface* between the immaterial and the physical realms.**

The actual point of interface can only be inferred. Within the brain, innate intelligence's *intent* to organize a specific tissue cell's response, which is immaterial, becomes imbedded in a newly formed nerve impulse, which is physical. This event cannot be interfered with, because it is not a "process" requiring time. It simply happens at the moment of energy transformation. Thus we conclude that such forces are *created perfect* ("100% force created"). As soon as they come into being, and begin to be transmitted, they can be interfered with, since transmission is a physical process that does take time.

STEP 7: Mental Impulse[61]

The seventh step in the Normal Complete Cycle is the *Mental Impulse.* This is the name given to the specific type of force created (or assembled) by the body's innate intelligence in the innate brain. A mental impulse is aptly named. It is *mental* because the source of the information (the forun) in the force is the body's innate intelligence in the *mental* realm. It is an *impulse* because the physical energy that carries the forun is a nerve impulse, generated by a neuron in the innate brain.

At the moment of its creation, as the immaterial message is embedded in the physical packet of energy, the mental impulse is presumed to be perfect. It has not yet existed physically for any time in which interference could happen to it. It is located in the brain and represents the living link between the intent of the body's

[60] *Ibid.* Art. 54, p. 23
[61] *Ibid.* Art. 59, p. 29

innate intelligence to cause a specific organized adaptive response in the body's matter, and the expression of that intent as adaptive action.

It is created in a particular neuron, which will allow the body's innate intelligence to target that particular mental impulse for a particular tissue cell of the innate body. In fact, which neuron the body's innate intelligence uses to create a particular mental impulse may be considered a significant aspect of the information said to be contained in that mental impulse. We can further speculate that, just as the informational content of a letter is embedded in its specific shape and position within a word, so might the informational content of a mental impulse be embedded in its frequency, intensity and the timing of its creation in the brain.

In any event, the creation of a specific mental impulse by the body's innate intelligence in a specific neuron at a specific moment in the body's functioning is nothing more or less than a specific message that the body's innate intelligence intends to send to the body. The message is one bit of the information necessary to direct the body's subsequent functioning one cell or cell group at a time. Of course, it is philosophically critical to remember that the body's innate intelligence, acting through the innate brain, actually creates millions of mental impulses at any one moment in time. It *can do so* because the body's innate intelligence is immaterial, infinite and perfect, and operates through all brain cells continuously. In the physical realm, the structure of the brain is sufficiently complex to allow for the creation of a vast number of mental impulses simultaneously (see *Step 16* below).

> We can further speculate that, just as the informational content of a letter is embedded in its specific shape and position within a word, so might the informational content of a mental impulse be embedded in its frequency, intensity and the timing of its creation in the brain.

STEP 8: Propulsion[62]

The eighth step of the Normal Complete Cycle is *Propulsion*. In Stephenson's *Chiropractic Textbook*, there is a discussion concerning the concept that a mental impulse, being created in the innate brain, must be propelled forth to travel over the appropriate nerve fiber to the appropriate peripheral innate body cell that is its intended destination.

More recently, our understanding of the evocation of a nerve impulse (an action potential along the axonal membrane) would suggest that the propulsion of a newly created mental impulse is an unnecessary concept. Rather, its propagation along the nerve axon is inherent in the mechanism of its generation.

[62] *Ibid*. Art. 60, p. 30

In any event, once created in a neuron, a mental impulse will commence to travel efferently along the axon of that neuron, which is designed by the body's innate intelligence as the appropriate conducting medium for this particular type of biological force. This also correctly implies that a mental impulse is a *conducted* force, carrying its information in a form of energy that necessarily travels along a material pathway.

STEP 9: Efferent Nerve[63]

The ninth step of the Normal Complete Cycle is the *Efferent Nerve*. The mental impulses created in the innate brain are conducted along a network of physical pathways, commonly referred to as the *nerve system,* designed by the body's innate intelligence and formed within the body's structure for the purpose of conducting the nerve impulses to specific target cells. Much of innate intelligence's ability to send specific messages to specific, specialized tissue cells is created by the specificity of the fibers and connections of the nerve system.

In this respect, the information transmission system of a living human body is analogous to a telephone system. To communicate among different, specialized members of a community, information can be *broadcast,* by way of a radio transmitter, or *specifically targeted* to specific individuals by way of personalized messages over a telephone system. Similarly, the body's innate intelligence can *broadcast* generalized adaptive messages non-specifically to large numbers of tissue cells by way of a hormonal message secreted into the blood circulatory system, or *send* individualized adaptive messages *specifically* to individual tissue cells over the nerve system. Both the hormonal and the neuronal communication systems are mechanisms to create and transmit regulating forces among the body's tissue cells. In fact, they are closely related to each other, with many of the neurotransmitters of the nerve system also serving in the role of hormonal messengers. However, they are still fundamentally distinguishable from each other by comparison between a hormone's slow, generalized effect on the body's adaptive responses and a mental impulse's rapid, specific effect.

In considering any one mental impulse, we can define its *efferent nerve* as the specific pathway along which that mental impulse is transmitted from the innate brain cell that assembled it to the specific innate body cell whose actions it is intended to influence. This pathway will usually consist of several neurons, their synaptic connections and the neuro-cellular junction at the peripheral terminus of the pathway. While this is conceptually easy to describe, the physical actuality of the efferent nerve system is almost inconceivably complex, as it allows for the transmission of forces created within billions of neurons to literally trillions of peripheral tissue cells.

[63] *Ibid.* Art. 61, p. 31

STEP 10: Transmission[64] (Step 2 of the Simple Cycle)

The tenth step of the Normal Complete Cycle is *Transmission*. This step constitutes the central or focal point of the process of adaptability as far as the chiropractic profession is concerned. The *transmission* to which it refers is the *actual, physical movement* of a mental impulse *from the innate brain cell* that the body's innate intelligence used to assemble it, *to the tissue cell* of the innate body that the body's innate intelligence intends to cause to respond adaptively.

> **The physical actuality of the efferent nerve system is almost inconceivably complex.**

Therefore, it comes as no surprise that Stephenson uses this step of the Normal Complete Cycle as the second step of his more streamlined Simple Cycle.

The thing that is being transmitted is the physical energy of the nerve impulse. Current theories concerning how this form of energy propagates through nerve tissue explain it as a surface disturbance of the balance of electrolytes across the cell membrane of the neuron. This electrochemical polarity reversal tends to self-propagate toward the cell body along one of a neuron's dendrites and away from the cell body along the neuron's axon.

A nerve impulse can also cross from one neuron to another in an efferent nerve pathway. This happens across what is referred to as a *synapse*. At this type of juncture between neurons, a propagating nerve impulse, arriving at the end of the neuron's axon, will cause the release of specific chemicals, called *neurotransmitters*, from the very terminus of the axon. These neurotransmitters then diffuse across the very narrow gap between the axonal end of this neuron and the dendritic end of the next neuron. Upon arriving at the cell membrane of the subsequent neuron on the other side of the synapse, the neurotransmitter stimulates it to initiate a second, self-propagating nerve impulse in this second neuron. In this manner, a mental impulse can and does move from one neuron to the next.

Transmission, as a step of the Normal Complete Cycle, implies the entire process of a mental impulse moving from the *point of* its *creation* in the brain to the *point of* its *intended effect* at the peripheral tissue cell. Transmission, therefore, implies that the nerve impulse following a nerve pathway is the physical mechanism designed to carry an *adaptive message from the body's innate intelligence* from the brain to a specific tissue cell or group of tissue cells.

The body's innate intelligence organizes the brain, the efferent nerve system and the peripheral tissue cells as an integrated system, designed to function via the normal creation, transmission and expression of these particular forces. Even the hormonal system, innate intelligence's other, related system of regulation and control, is itself controlled and regulated by mental impulses created in the brain, transmitted over efferent nerves and expressed by the function of the hormone-

[64] *Ibid.* Art. 62, p. 31

producing glands.

The transmission of adaptive information embedded in efferent nerve impulses is central to the overall functioning of the body. Therefore it is logical to infer that *any interference* to the normal and proper transmission of these efferent nerve messages would disturb and render less efficient the functions these messages are intended to cause. If we have evidence and/or believe that vertebral subluxations can and necessarily do cause interference to the transmission of mental impulses, then it is necessary to conclude that vertebral subluxations disturb and render less efficient the adaptive functioning of the body. From this simple, logical syllogism, the chiropractic profession takes its central clinical objective – to locate, analyze and correct any and all vertebral subluxations in any and all persons.

The transmission of adaptive information embedded in efferent nerve impulses is central to the overall functioning of the body.

Another necessary conclusion of this logical syllogism is that the mechanism whereby a vertebral mal-juxtaposition may produce an alteration of the conductive properties of nerve tissue and, consequently, interference to the transmission of the mental impulse, is probably the single most central scientific question to arise from this philosophic model of health. This question must necessarily focus on the physical alteration of the nerve impulse, since we can *only infer* that inappropriate distortions of the physical energy of a force will alter the *message* in that force. However, this is a strong logical inference to make, and we have many examples from our own experience on which to draw.

The message itself can, ultimately, only be interpreted by the intelligence that receives that message, i.e. the innate intelligence of the tissue cell receiving the mental impulse. Therefore, the actual existence of interference to that message can only truly be known to the body's innate intelligence, through its awareness of the reception of a distorted message by the innate body cell.

We can, however, validly infer the existence of interference to the adaptive message in a mental impulse two ways. We can look for evidence of factors known to alter the propagation of a particular form of energy, in this case the nerve impulse. We can also look for evidence of an alteration of the expected expression of a force. Since the expected expression of a mental impulse is an adaptive response on the part of the body, we can interpret a diminution of that adaptive vigor as evidence of interference to the messages embedded within the adaptive mental impulses. Chiropractic techniques for the location and analysis of vertebral subluxation regularly employ both of these approaches.

Finally, *transmission,* as Step 10 of the Normal Complete Cycle, implies that the mental impulse travels from the innate brain cell to the innate body cell successfully, i.e. *without interference*. If interference occurs at this point of the Normal Complete Cycle, it would no longer be a Normal Complete Cycle. Instead, it (the interference) would initiate a cycle of incoordination or *dis-ease*.[65]

STEP 11: Tissue Cell[66]

The eleventh step of the Normal Complete Cycle is *Tissue Cell*. The tissue cell referred to in this step is the *innate body cell*, which may be defined as a tissue cell that receives mental impulses from the *innate mind* to direct and coordinate its function. This may be any type of tissue cell designed by the body's innate intelligence to accomplish a particular adaptive function for the good of the whole body.

Which specific tissue cell receives the mental impulse determines to a great extent what function that mental impulse will initiate. The message in a mental impulse appears to be able to tell a tissue cell when to function and for how long, but the actual nature of that function will be determined *not* by the mental impulse, but by the structure of the tissue cell expressing the mental impulse. As Stephenson puts it, "It *(the tissue cell)* may have many functions but that one for which it is built, and which it does coordinately or cooperatively for the benefit and welfare of the other tissues of the body, is the function mentioned in this cycle."[67]

While we say that the tissue cell receives and expresses the mental impulse, it is actually the body's innate intelligence expressing itself through that tissue cell that receives, interprets and responds to the mental impulse. Matter cannot receive and interpret information, any more than it can create and send information. But since the body's innate intelligence constitutes the *immaterial component* of any tissue cell that receives a mental impulse, as well as the tissue cell that sends it (the *innate brain cell*), tissue cells can *respond* to mental impulses, as well as send them. Another way of saying this is that, if the tissue cell were not alive, and therefore not expressing its own innate intelligence as living activity, that tissue cell would react differently to the force of a mental impulse than a living cell would. It would react to the energetic component of the force, as any matter must, but it would not be able to *respond adaptively* to the forun, the message being sent to it. Again, Stephenson puts it very succinctly when he says, "Therefore, each tissue cell is an organism and, therefore, there is intelligence in

> **Every tissue cell is an independently living organism in its own right, surviving by adapting to its own environment, namely the body of which it is a part.**

[65] *Ibid*. Art. 122, p. 82 *ff*.
[66] *Ibid*. Art. 63, p. 32
[67] *Ibid*.

it. It is absolutely essential that the units composing the body be of this nature *(alive and healthy themselves)*, else Innate could not control them."[68]

The concept of the tissue cell in this step also denotes a specific adaptive tool, built and maintained by the body's innate intelligence to function as a co-ordinated part of the whole organism. Neurologically regulated organisms are necessarily multi-cellular organisms. Multi-cellular organisms work on the principle of specialization of tasks. In other words, even though each tissue cell is an independently living organism in its own right, surviving by adapting to its own environment (namely the body of which it is a part), its particular structure allows it to perform a particular kind of activity that serves not just its own needs, but the needs of the organism as a whole. This is its special task, which will be discussed below as its *function.*

STEP 12: Reception[69]

The twelfth step of the Normal Complete Cycle is *Reception.* This step simply denotes that, after its transmission over the efferent nerve pathway, a mental impulse arrives at the tissue cell or cells of the innate body that it is intended to cause to respond adaptively.

Calling this step reception rather than "arrival" implies that, as the mental impulse arrives, there is also an action on the part of the innate body cell. It physically and temporally *receives* the mental impulse, but, since a mental impulse is also a *force,* it must necessarily also **respond to** that mental impulse. This must necessarily be considered a *response,* and not just a reaction, because the tissue cell's response to the mental impulse isn't passive, as if it were a lump of clay. Rather, because the tissue cell itself is a living thing in its own right, it will make an active, adaptive response.

The innate body cell that receives the mental impulse *must* respond. Remember that a mental impulse is a force, composed of energy and adaptive information. While we are concerned with the quality and significance of the information the body's innate intelligence has embedded in the mental impulse, the energy of the nerve impulse carrying the adaptive message is equally significant. It is this energy that compels action on the part of the innate body cell. This is why a mental impulse is an *impulse;* because it impels the tissue cell into action. The adaptive message only tells the cell when, how much and/or what kind of action to undertake.

---

[68]*Ibid.* Art. 85, p. 52
[69]*Ibid.* Art. 79, p. 46

CHAPTER 13

The Tissue Cell's Response to the Mental Impulse

"If a bear starts to chase us, I'm taking off as fast as I can."
"Who are you kidding? You can't run faster than a bear."
"I don't have to. I just need to run faster than you."

ANONYMOUS

The next four steps of the Normal Complete Cycle, *Physical Personification, Expression, Function* and *Coordination,* which are the final four steps of the efferent side of the cycle, all describe what a tissue cell does in response to its reception of the mental impulse. As you consider these four steps, remember that they are all describing different aspects of the same action, the adaptive response of an innate body cell to the message in a mental impulse.

STEP 13: Physical Personification[70]

The thirteenth step of the Normal Complete Cycle is *Physical Personification.* This step means exactly what its name implies; that something which wasn't physical before becomes manifested physically. At this point we may ask ourselves what remains to be physically manifested. The answer is that the forun, innate intelligence's bit of adaptive information, created in the mental ream and embedded in the mental impulse, has yet to be physically manifested. It is the forun that is physically personified in this step.

The forun is information; more specifically it is adaptive information, which means that it is the aspect of a mental impulse that determines *how* the energy will affect matter's motion. Thus, when the mental impulse affects the tissue cell's motion, (or the tissue cell responds to the mental impulse), the forun (the adaptive message) becomes physically personified as the tissue cell's adaptive motion.[71]

One crucial element of this concept is that physical personification will occur *no matter what the information in the mental impulse is!* This means that, although in the Normal Complete Cycle we are considering the effect of a mental impulse transmitted without interference, were there to be interference to the transmission of a mental impulse, there would *still be physical personification by the tissue cell.* It would just be the physical manifestation of a now distorted, less than perfect

---

[70] *Ibid.* Art. 80, p. 46
[71] *Ibid.* Art. 330, p. 254

message, and the resulting motion on the part of the tissue cell would be less than perfectly adaptive. In fact, the tissue cell's motion would be incoordinated, rather than adaptive, *dis-eased* rather than *at ease.*

Were there to be interference to the transmission of a mental impulse, the tissue cell's motion would be incoordinated, rather than adaptive, *dis-eased* rather than *at ease.*

The physical personification of a perfect forun by a healthy innate body cell is one small but totally crucial element of the overall process of adaptation. It is one bit of the manifestation of the total physical coordination called health (See *Step 16* below). It is the physical adaptation that follows the intellectual adaptation which the body's innate intelligence makes.

STEP 14: Expression[72]

The fourteenth step of the Normal Complete Cycle is *Expression.* This step, as an aspect of the tissue cell's response to a mental impulse, refers to the most basic idea of the duality between intelligence and matter. If intelligence, whether referred to as universal or innate, represents the universe's *intent to organize itself,* then matter's organization, its specific patterns of interrelated motion, represents *the expression of that intent.* Thus *expression* means the successful translation of intelligence's intent into action. For this reason, it also serves as the third step of the Simple Cycle, completing the efferent side, and leading to the afferent steps.

Expression is subtly different than Physical Personification, the previous step of the Normal Complete Cycle. Consider the following illustration. If someone asks you to "dance a jig," but he or she mumbles, or perhaps your ears are full of wax and you don't hear the instructions clearly, so you "lance a pig" instead, your action *is* the physical personification of the message you received, **but not** of the message being sent. In other words, it does not express *the intent* of the person sending the message. However, if that person, speaking clearly, asks you to "dance a jig," and you, hearing clearly, dance the jig as requested, your action is not only the *physical personification of the message* you received, but also the *expression of the intent* of the person in sending the message in the first place. It is the same with a tissue cell receiving a mental impulse. When a tissue cell receives a mental impulse and responds *adaptively,* this actually represents the *expression* of the body's innate intelligence on *three distinct levels.*

First, the physical personification of the forun, the message in the mental impulse, is the expression of the intent of the body's innate intelligence in creating the mental impulse in the first place. In creating a forun and assembling a mental impulse in the innate brain, the body's innate intelligence has an intelligent purpose; namely to send an adaptive message to a particular tissue cell. It is

[72]*Ibid.* Art. 81, p. 48

sending this message because the body's innate intelligence knows that the over-all good of the body requires that tissue cell's adaptive response (function) at that moment in time. At this level, the tissue cell's appropriate adaptive response to the mental impulse expresses the intent of the body's innate intelligence *in creating the mental impulse in the first place.*

Secondly, the physical personification of a mental impulse is the expression of the intent of the body's innate intelligence in building and maintaining that particular tissue cell as a healthy living thing in its own right. Only a living, healthy tissue cell *can respond adaptively* to a mental impulse. Thus, the adaptive response denotes the expression of the body's innate intelligence through the five "signs of life" of that tissue cell. Closely related to this level of expression is the fact that the body's innate intelligence anatomically designs an innate body cell to be able to receive and respond to mental impulses. Thus the adaptive response also denotes the expression of the body's innate intelligence in *designing a receiver* for the messages it sends via the innate mind.

Finally, the physical personification of a mental impulse is the expression of the innate intelligence of the tissue cell in receiving, properly interpreting and correctly responding to the message in the mental impulse. When it is created in the innate brain, a mental impulse is an internal biological force, carrying con-structive, adaptive information to the tissue cell, information that is constructive in terms of what is good for the *whole body.* But if we consider it from the innate body cell's perspective, a mental impulse is an *environmental* (external) force. And while the forun in the mental impulse is certainly constructive to the whole body, it may not necessarily contribute to the good or well-being of that particular tissue cell itself. The tissue cell must be able to discriminate that the forun should be physically personified, even if it is harmful to that individual tissue cell's own chances of survival. We must infer that the body's innate intelligence, acting within that tissue cell, can decide to act for the good of the whole body over the good of the individual tissue cell. Thus, the tissue cell's adaptive response expresses the intent of the body's innate intelligence in *meeting the needs of the whole organism at the level of the action of the individual cell.*

Finally, whereas a mental impulse can be *physical personified* as either health or, consequent to interference, as incoordination, the *expression* of a mental im-pulse *always* implies a healthy, adaptive response. This is simply because any *in-terference* to the transmission of a mental impulse would lessen the clarity of the information that represents the intent of the body's innate intelligence in creat-ing the mental impulse in the first place. The message representing innate intelli-gence's intent is garbled, which necessarily reduces or eliminates the *expression* of that intent when the mental impulse is actually personified (its information trans-

The tissue cell's response to a mental impulse expresses the body's *innate intelligence* in three different ways:

It expresses the intent of the body's innate intelligence in creating the mental impulse in the first place.

It expresses the intent of the body's innate intelligence in designing a receiver for the messages it sends.

It expresses the intent of the body's innate intelligence in meeting the needs of the whole organism at the level of the action of the individual cell.

lated into action). A damaged or unfit tissue cell could also lessen expression, even in the absence of interference. The message may get through without distortion, but the damaged or unfit tissue cell is expressing the body's innate intelligence *within itself* less than perfectly and is thereby *unable to respond fully* to the mental impulse. This would not be dis-ease, however, since it is not the result of interference. It would be the destructive effect of tissue cell *trauma*.

STEP 15: Function[73]

The fifteenth step of the Normal Complete Cycle is *Function*. This denotes the *useful task or job* the tissue cell does *for the good of the whole body*. Function differs from the internal, metabolic activities a tissue cell must carry out to express its own life. In order to be a living thing, a muscle cell does not have to contract. It only has to assimilate, eliminate, grow, reproduce (as necessary) and adapt. But a muscle cell is *designed* to contract. It does so not for its own benefit, but simply because the body's innate intelligence formed it in such a way that, when it receives a mental impulse, *it must contract*. The body's innate intelligence knows that this tissue cell's contraction is not necessarily useful or meaningful to the tissue cell itself, but is useful in meeting the needs of the whole body, and is *only* meaningful in the context of the needs of the whole body.

Every tissue cell that receives mental impulses has the extra ability to do some unique task that relates not to its own needs, but to the needs of the whole organism of which it is a part. This unique task is that cell's *function*. Examples abound. Islets of Langerhans cells don't need all the insulin they synthesize, but the rest of body does need that insulin. RBCs neither need nor utilize the oxygen they transport, but the body needs for that oxygen to be transported. Some cells die performing their function, and others must even *die in order to perform their function*. For example, macrophages don't need to engulf and digest foreign bacteria to survive. Actually, it often kills them to do so, yet they do engulf and digest foreign bacteria *for the good of the whole body*. Epidermal cells, which form the water-resistant outer surface of the skin, don't even become functional *until* they die and become keratinized. Cells such as these are often not directly connected

[73] *Ibid.* Art. 82, p. 48

to the efferent nerve network, and thus are not technically innate body cells. Nonetheless, they express the body's innate intelligence in their own activities and have important functions to perform, as well.

Function, as a step of the Normal Complete Cycle, denotes that expression is *individualized* for each tissue cell as its individual, characteristic *type of adaptive motion*. This unique type of motion is its function, and its function is the expression of innate

Function denotes the useful task or job the tissue cell does for the good of the whole body.

intelligence within the structure of that particular tissue cell. While it is the mental impulse it receives that *causes* an innate body cell to function, it is the tissue cell's specific structure that *determines what its function will actually be*.

Note that a tissue cell's characteristic, function-determining structure is *also* an expression of the body's innate intelligence. All tissue cells of a living organism have the same genetic code and differ in structure only through the process of "differentiation." Differentiation simply denotes variation in cell structure within a developing embryo. It results from the expression of different elements of the DNA code within differentiating cells. This is a living process and therefore it represents the expression of the body's innate intelligence through the matter of the embryo.

Expression denotes how a tissue cell, responding to a mental impulse, serves the body's innate intelligence. Function denotes how that tissue cell's response serves the interests of the whole body. While we have noted that a tissue cell's function does not necessarily serve its own interests directly, it is also worth noting that tissue cells that do not perform their proper functions, for whatever reason, tend to atrophy and die. From this we can certainly infer that the act of functioning for the good of the whole organism does return some vital benefit to the individual tissue cell itself. We also see parallels to this in our own functioning as parts of organizational structures larger than ourselves, such as families, communities and nations. Even though service to a larger whole may involve sacrifices, it returns rewards to the individual that cannot be earned in the context of the individual acting alone.

STEP 16: Coordination[74]

The sixteenth and last efferent step of the Normal Complete Cycle is *Coordination*. This step denotes the harmonious interaction (ease) of *all tissue cells* working in coordination with each other for the good of the whole organism. For conceptual simplicity, the Normal Complete Cycle looks at the process of adaptation from the perspective of the body's innate intelligence creating adap-

---

[74] *Ibid.* Art. 85, p. 51

tive responses one cell at a time. The reality of the situation, however, is that the response of each tissue cell can only be truly adaptive if its actions are *harmoniously blended* with the simultaneous actions *of all other tissue cells.*

Up to this point, each step of the Normal Complete Cycle has recounted what the body's innate intelligence has done relative to the proper role of each cell (innate brain cell, efferent nerve cell, innate body cell) in the creation, transmission and expression of one mental impulse. *Coordination,* as the final efferent step of the Normal Complete Cycle, denotes that the body's innate intelligence must necessarily control and regulate the activities of countless innate body cells *simultaneously,* through the creation of countless mental impulses in the (literally) billions of innate brain cells of a single living human being (for example).

The body's innate intelligence is capable of performing this volume of intelligent creation because it is immaterial, inexhaustible and infinite in its capacity to create information. It is a sufficient cause not only for all the organization of the individual living organism, but for *all living organisms and all other organization of the universe at the same time.* As we remember from our definitions, the body's innate intelligence is just universal intelligence under a different name. The name "innate intelligence" denotes that this infinite, perfect organizing intelligence is being expressed through the matter and activities of a particular living thing.

How much attention does the body's innate intelligence devote to meeting the body's needs? It will devote all that is necessary from its infinite, inexhaustible capacity.

Having said this, it is worth considering that, in the ability of the body's innate intelligence's to control and coordinate the activities of so many tissue cells, all directed toward one overall adaptive purpose, we can begin to *see and appreciate* what Stephenson actually means when he characterizes the body's innate intelligence as being infinite and perfect. How much attention does the body's innate intelligence, literally the intelligence of the entire universe brought to bear on the organizational needs of a specific living organism, devote to meeting those needs? It will devote all that is necessary from its infinite, inexhaustible capacity.[75]

Coordination is the name we give to the expression of *all* the "bits of attention" (foruns) the body's innate intelligence pays in creating *all* the mental impulses it creates at any one moment in time. It is actually coordination, in the larger perspective of all the body's cells, tissues, organs and organ systems interacting, that is the *ease,* the *overall physical adaptation,* indeed, the *health* of a living organism.

---

[75] Principle 8 – The amount of intelligence for any given amount of matter is 100%, and is always proportional to its requirements, p. 78 above

CHAPTER 14

The Afferent Side of the Normal Complete Cycle

"Cheshire Puss," she began, rather timidly, as she did not at all know whether it would like the name: however it only grinned a little wider. "Come, it's pleased so far," thought Alice and she went on. "Would you tell me, please, which way I ought to go from here?"

"That depends a good deal on where you want to get to," said the Cat.

"I don't much care where—" said Alice.

"Then it doesn't matter which way you go," said the Cat.

LEWIS CARROLL (1865)

STEP 17: Coordination[76]

The seventeenth step of the Normal Complete Cycle is also called *Coordination,* as is *Step 16* above. In fact, this step simply represents "turning the corner" from efferent to afferent. The last step of the efferent side of the Normal Complete Cycle becomes the first step of the afferent side. In other words, coordination, the harmonious interaction (ease) of *all tissue cells* interacting with each other for the good of the whole organism, can be viewed two ways. We can consider it as the *end result* of the efferent activities of the body's innate intelligence expressing itself, i.e. the efferent side of the Normal Complete Cycle. But it is also the *starting point* for innate intelligence's awareness of the state of the body, and therefore its awareness of the needs of the body, that will drive the next iteration of the cycle, i.e. the afferent side of the Normal Complete Cycle.

In looking at coordination from the afferent aspect of this process, we also begin to look at the whole process in afferent terms. This means that, from now to the end of the Normal Complete Cycle, we are considering the relationship between the matter of the body (i.e. its particular, momentary "condition" and the forces that create and influence the current state of its organization) and the body's innate intelligence. This is what "afferent" refers to in the Normal Complete Cycle; namely the flow of information from the matter of the physical body back to the body's innate intelligence.

Note that this philosophic concept of what "afferent" refers to is subtly different than the physiological meaning of "afferent." Physiologically, "afferent" usually refers to the flow of neurological impulses from the peripheral tissues back to the brain. However, this is based on the assumption that the biological

[76] Stephenson's *Chiropractic Textbook,* 1948 ed., Art. 86, p. 52

The body's innate intelligence is not "located" in the brain; it is the immaterial component of *all of the matter* of the living organism.

duality is the brain and the body. In chiropractic, we are reasoning from the assumption that the basic biological duality is between the body's innate intelligence and the body's substance. Therefore, the afferent flow of information is not from innate body to innate brain, but from the organism's physical matter to its immaterial innate intelligence. Information does not need to go to the brain to "get to" the body's innate intelligence. The body's innate intelligence is not "located" in the brain; it is the immaterial component of *all of the matter* of the living organism.

There certainly exists a *physical afferent flow* of nerve impulses over and/or through *physical afferent nerves* within a living organism, which the body's innate intelligence creates for the proper functioning of the educated mind, as is discussed in what Stephenson's *Chiropractic Textbook* calls the "Special Sense Cycle." This, however, has to do with the body's innate intelligence using the brain as an information processing organ. The role of the brain as an organ for collecting, storing and processing information, and the relationship between these functions and the expression of the body's innate intelligence, are discussed as a separate, though related, topic called the "Inter-Brain Cycle"[77] in several articles in Stephenson's *Chiropractic Textbook*.

Coordination, as the first step of the afferent side of the Normal Complete Cycle, takes into consideration the harmonious interaction of *all* tissue cells interacting with each other for the good of the whole organism. This means that, from this point forward in the Normal Complete Cycle, we are considering the functions of *all* body cells, not just the cells of the innate body, but the efferent nerve cells and the cells of the innate brain as well. The Normal Complete Cycle looks at innate intelligence's *control of the body* at the level of the nerve system's role as a regulatory mechanism. On the other hand, it looks at innate intelligence's *awareness of the body* at all levels, from the atomic and molecular to the cellular to the intercellular (whole organism) levels.

STEP 18: Tissue Cell[78]

The eighteenth step of the Normal Complete Cycle is *Tissue Cell*. Again, this can simply be considered "turning the corner" from efferent to afferent consideration. In the efferent side of the Normal Complete Cycle, we considered the tissue cell as the recipient and ultimate expresser of internal biological forces, particularly the metal impulse. On the afferent side of Normal Complete Cycle, we will consider the tissue cell as the starting point of innate intelligence's aware-

---

[77] *Ibid.* Art. 112, p. 74; Art. 319, p. 242 ff.
[78] *Ibid.* Art. 87, p. 52

ness of the state and needs of the body. From this perspective, the *final effect* of efferent function (the tissue cell receiving and expressing forces as alterations to its motions) becomes an *initial cause* of afferent function (the tissue cell's altered motions informing the awareness of the body's innate intelligence.)

It is also necessary to consider that the internal, biological forces created, transmitted and expressed by the tissue cells *are not the only forces influencing the motion* of the body's matter. At this point in the Normal Complete Cycle, the effects of any and all *environmental forces* that impinge on the living organism must also be considered. These will consist primarily of forces coming from outside the organism, i.e. from its *external* environment. On the other hand, forces introduced into the internal environment as waste products of tissue cell metabolism and function must also be considered. This perspective is crucial because the actual state of the body's matter, of which the body's innate intelligence must ultimately be aware, always reflects the net effect of *all forces* acting on that matter.

STEP 19: Vibration[79]

The nineteenth step of the Normal Complete Cycle is *Vibration*. "Vibration" is used in the Normal Complete Cycle to indicate any and all *types and/or levels of motion* in the matter of the physical body. In looking at vibration as the starting point for innate intelligence's awareness of the current organization of the physical body, and its consequent analysis of the body's current needs, we can resolve vibration into three distinctly different, although closely interrelated, levels of specific motions. These include *physical vibration, metabolic vibration* and *functional vibration.*

Physical vibrations include those specific motions of matter at the level of its atomic and molecular organization. These vibrations are not unique motions of the matter in its role as a part of the living organism. Rather, these types of vibration are inherent to the organization of matter at its simplest levels (although some molecular vibrations are distinctive to the living processes of the organism.)

Neither the specific motions of the protons, neutrons and electrons that form oxygen and hydrogen atoms, nor the specific motions of the oxygen and hydrogen atoms that form water molecules, are given to that matter by the internal biological forces generated by living processes. Certainly, water that is part of a living organism will have these specific motions, but so will the water in a lake or an ice cube.

Metabolic vibrations include those specific motions of matter at the level of its organization as a living cell. In considering the tissue cell as the basic structural and functional unit of a typical, multi-cellular living organism, we can discern the

[79] *Ibid.* Art. 88, p. 53

existence of a great many specific motions of matter relative to the tissue cell's expression of innate intelligence at the cellular level. A tissue cell itself is a living thing. As such, its atoms and molecules are undergoing many specific living motions that are unique and characteristic to the cell's organization and survival.

Water that is a part of a living tissue cell has the physical vibrations of the water molecules, but also the metabolic vibration of being a component of the cell's cytoplasm (for example), or being formed by carbohydrate combustion in the Krebs cycle. These motions would be examples of metabolic vibrations. In fact, any motion of the tissue cell's matter in expressing its own signs of life, in assimilating, eliminating, growing, reproducing and adapting itself, would be considered metabolic vibrations.

Metabolic vibrations *are caused* by the internal biological forces created, transmitted and expressed within the confines of the tissue cell. They can also be influenced by the internal, biological forces created within the body, but external to the individual tissue cell. Generally, the effects of hormones on tissue cells are examples of this. However, in the case of extra-cellular hormonal influences, the forces still have to be assimilated and adapted by the body's innate intelligence acting within the tissue cell itself. Any changes in the cell's metabolic activities in response to these types of forces would also be metabolic vibrations.

> The *functional vibration* of an innate brain cell would be its motion in assembling a mental impulse; of an efferent nerve cell, the motion of the passage of the mental impulse along its membrane.

Functional vibrations are those specific motions of a tissue cell that contribute not necessarily to the tissue cell's own survival, but to the overall adaptation and survival of the whole living organism. The actual movement of the contraction of a muscle cell, both internally and externally, would be an example of a functional vibration, as would the synthesis and excretion of a hormonal protein molecule from a glandular cell. The functional vibration of an innate brain cell would be its motion in assembling a mental impulse; of an efferent nerve cell, the passage of the mental impulse along its membrane.

In the innate body, *functional vibrations* are the tissue cell's response to the mental impulse. Thus, we can say that the *structure* of the tissue cell *determines* what its functional vibrations will be, but that the *mental impulse* actually causes the tissue cell to undergo its particular functional vibration.

As we know from our earlier discussion of matter's properties and actions, the specific motions of matter at any and all levels of vibration, which determine the specific relationships among the material parts of any organized thing, determine the actual, particular state of organization of that thing. Applying this concept to the levels of vibration in living organisms as described above, we can say that the **whole living organism is healthy** when all of its parts (tissue cells) are constructed from matter with the optimum *physical vibrations* (made out of the 'right stuff'), are maintaining themselves in a state of optimum *metabolic vibration* (the cells themselves are internally healthy), and are all performing harmonious, coordinated physical motions, called *functions,* which express the intent of its own innate intelligence and meet the needs of the organism as a whole, over and above the needs of the individual cells themselves.

Such a "dynamic state of harmonic vibration at all levels of motion" expresses both the intent of the organism's innate intelligence in bringing those physical parts together as an integrated whole structure, and its intention to maintain that state of vibration through the adaptation of potentially *destructive* environmental forces into *constructive* internal, biological forces. If, on the other hand, the body is traumatized, it is in a state of inharmonious, uncoordinated physical vibration brought about by the effects of external, environmental forces that change the body's material motions in ways that do not reflect the intent of the body's innate intelligence. If it is incoordinated *(dis-eased),* it is in a state of inharmonious, uncoordinated physical vibration brought about by interference to the transmission and expression of those internal biological forces that where created, initially, to change the body's material motions adaptively. In any event, health, trauma and dis-ease are all *states of vibration* of the living organism's physical matter.

> **Health, trauma and dis-ease are all states of vibration of the living organism's physical matter.**

STEP 20: Impressions of Vibrations[80]

The twentieth step of the Normal Complete Cycle, which is also the first *afferent* step (Step 4) of the Simple Cycle, is *Impressions of Vibrations.* In chiropractic philosophy, the term *impression* denotes the meaningful message that any and every vibration in the physical realm communicates to the body's innate intelligence in the mental realm. This is a concept necessitated by the following line of reasoning.

Efferently, in order for the *immaterial creativity* of life (the body's innate intelligence) to affect the *physical activity* of the matter of a living organism (its organization), there must be a link between the two that can go from immaterial to material. Information (the forun) provides just such a link. Information, which is *potential form,* comes from intelligence, is communicated to matter (via force), and is interpreted by that matter to become the form of its response (adaptive motion).

Similarly, on the afferent side, in order for the *physical activity* of the matter

[80] *Ibid.* Art. 89, p. 54

of a living organism (its organization) to affect the *immaterial creativity* of life (the body's innate intelligence), there must also be a link between the two that can go, in this case, from the material realm to the immaterial realm. The concept of the *impressions of vibrations* provides just such an afferent link.

Why should we use the term "impression" and what do we mean by it? Is it related to our use of the term *information?* On the one hand, it is similar to the concept of information, simply because an impression, like an informational forum, can cross the interface between the material and the immaterial realms.

An *impression* is "the meaningful message a physical vibration sends to the Mental Realm."

On the other hand, it would not do to use the term "information" itself. We consider the efferent influence (coming from intelligence to matter) to be *potential form* (information), because matter can have form, *but not awareness.* Analogously, we would have to consider the afferent influence (going from matter to intelligence) to be *potential awareness,* because intelligence can have awareness, *but not form.* Thus we are left with the question of what to call a "unit of potential awareness." In this case, Stephenson's use of the term *impression* certainly seems to be conceptually accurate and therefore appropriate.

Consider the following analogy as a crude approximation of the afferent relationship between vibrations in the physical realm (the actual organized motions of matter) and innate intelligence's awareness of organization in the mental realm. You are walking down a smooth, sandy beach, and you see an impression in the sand in front of you, which you recognize as a human footprint. You know that the footprint in the sand is not the same thing as the foot that left it there. As a matter of fact, the foot and the footprint exist within entirely different media, and the footprint can exist there even though the foot is no longer there. If you consider this situation carefully, you will also realize that what you are seeing isn't even actually a "footprint" *per se;* it is simply an impression of something that happened within a realm of activity adjacent to the sand. In fact, the identification of that impression as a "footprint" is actually the result of your intelligent awareness and analysis of the impression left in the sand.

Similarly, we can conceive of the relationship between a physical vibration and the body's innate intelligence acting in the mental realm. Physical vibration happens and has form in the physical realm. At the same time, the mental realm exists, different from but "adjacent to" the physical realm at all points. Each and every physical vibration leaves a "footprint," which is its corresponding *impression* in the mental realm. And, just as each footprint is separate and distinct, and corresponds to the form of the foot that left it in the sand, so each impression is separate and distinct and corresponds to the form of the physical vibration that creates that impression in the mental realm.

Thus, an impression is "the meaningful message a physical vibration sends to the Mental Realm." And, like a footprint on a beach, the impression exists separate from the vibration that creates it and/or the intelligence that perceives and interprets its meaning.

STEP 21: Afferent Nerve[81]

The twenty-first step of the Normal Complete Cycle is *Afferent Nerve*. This step, together with Step 22 *(Transmission)* and Step 23 *(Brain Cell),* constitute the most confusing and least well thought out parts of the Normal Complete Cycle, as it is presented in Stephenson's *Chiropractic Textbook*. The main problem arises from the unclear overlapping between the physical afferent *Special Sense Cycle,* involving the educated brain/mind, and the immaterial awareness of the body's innate intelligence in response to the impressions it receives of all the vibrations of the physical matter of the body.

The special sense functions of the educated brain/mind involve the brain's response to physical *special sense impulses,* created within peripheral *special sense receptor cells* (specialized neurons), transmitted over physical *afferent nerves* to the educated brain/mind, and the educated brain/mind's response to those physical forces. These special sense impulses form the basis for the educated brain/mind's "awareness" of the environment and certain aspects of the body itself.

Such educated (conscious) "awareness," however, is not the same as innate intelligence's total, perfect awareness of the matter through which it is being expressed. Rather, it is a physiological function of the brain as a living organ, and is therefore an *expression* of the body's innate intelligence, *not a direct action* of the body's innate intelligence itself. On the other hand, in the Normal Complete Cycle, we are examining innate intelligence's perfect (ideal) awareness of the body, which is called its "ideation."[82]

In light of the difference between the educated mind's special senses and innate intelligence's ideation (perfect awareness), the concept of the "afferent nerve" actually doesn't fit very well into the Normal Complete Cycle at all. In fact, it is probably more logically consistent to say that there is a material/immaterial *interface* between the physical realm and the mental realm, across which an impression travels from the physical vibration that creates it to the body's innate intelligence, which perceives and analyses it. This interface has been described as the theo-

The "pathway" between the physical and mental realms lies in their intimate, point for point adjacency as the two different but interdependent dimensions of being.

[81] *Ibid.* Art. 90, p. 55
[82] See *Step 28* below

retical afferent route,[83] although such a characterization may be unnecessarily mechanistic and confusing. In the final analysis, it would be more philosophically consistent and clearer if we simply noted that the "pathway" between the physical and mental realms lies in their intimate, point-for point adjacency as the two different but interdependent dimensions of being.

STEP 22: Transmission[84] (Afferent Transformation?)

The twenty-second step of the Normal Complete Cycle is *Transmission*. This step is also the fifth step of the Simple Cycle, representing *afferent transmission* from the tissue cell to the brain cell. Although our discussion below will involve some reinterpretation of what the concept of *afferent transmission* actually refers to, in the simplest sense, this step will still represent the concept that what happens to the body's matter must, ultimately, come back to the body's innate intelligence for interpretation.

Of course, it is immediately obvious that this step is conceived of and consequently named in relationship to the concept of the afferent nerve. However, it becomes inconsistent and confusing to call this process "transmission" if, in light of the discussion above, we *don't* consider the pathway to be the afferent nerve. Our understanding will be better served if we reserve the use of the term "transmission" to denote the physical process whereby a force moves through space and time from one point (point of creation) to another (point of intended expression). The use of the term "transmission" is further problematic because transmission, being a physical process, can be interfered with,[85] whereas the creation of impressions in the mental realm theoretically *cannot* be interfered with.

If we eliminate the concept that this step represents a true *transmission,* we are left with the question of what we should call the process whereby an impression "enters into" the mental realm. The solution becomes immediately clear, and the Normal Complete Cycle more internally consistent, if we consider the other point in the Normal Complete Cycle where this process of moving between the physical and the mental realms also occurs. When an immaterial forun (adaptive information) becomes associated with a bit of physical energy (the nerve impulse) to create a mental impulse, we call that process "transformation." The process whereby the immaterial meaning (the impression) of a physical vibration enters into the mental realm would certainly be a similar, though reversed, "transformation." To clarify this concept further, we could re-label the process of a forun transforming into a mental impulse as "Efferent Transformation"[86] and the process of the form of a physical vibration transforming into an immaterial

---

[83] *Ibid.* Art. 225, p.176
[84] *Ibid.* Art. 91, p. 57
[85] Principle 29 – There can be interference with the transmission of internal biological forces, p. 80 above
[86] See *Step 6* above

impression as "Afferent Transformation."

STEP 23: Brain Cell[87]

The twenty-third step of the Normal Complete Cycle is called *Brain Cell*. The description in Stephenson's *Chiropractic Textbook* indicates that this is to be considered the *innate brain cell*. Once again, and finally, this appears to be logically inconsistent. Here we have the final point of confusion and overlap between the physiology of special sense perception and the meta-physiology of innate intelligence's ideation (perfect awareness) of the body's state of organization. This step should be deleted from the conceptual flow of the Normal Complete Cycle. As per Stephenson's own definitions of innate brain cell and innate mind, there is no necessary afferent function of the innate mind (the innate brain actively expressing the body's innate intelligence). This simply derives from the philosophically non-rigorous and incorrect use of the terms "innate intelligence" and "innate mind" interchangeably. While this topic can only be completely explored and clarified within the context of a discussion of the *Inter-Brain Cycle,* suffice it to say that the body's innate intelligence does not carry out its own immaterial activities *from within the confines of* the innate brain. And it certainly could not *express* its own perfect awareness through the functioning of the innate mind, since ideation, to be perfect, must also be *immaterial*. The conclusion must be that innate intelligence's awareness and the activities that create it exist entirely in the immaterial mental realm.

> **Innate intelligence's awareness, and the activities that create it, exist entirely in the immaterial mental realm.**

STEP 24: Reception[88]

The twenty-fourth step of the Normal Complete Cycle is called *Reception.* Again, it is intuitively obvious that this step is a misdirected attempt to relate the immaterial process of awareness to the physical process of the special sense perception. We could stretch the concept and say that the impression "arrives" in the mental realm and the body's innate intelligence "receives" it. But this tends to confuse the idea that a physical vibration simply creates an impression in the mental realm.

On the other hand, if "reception" is understood as the concept that, as soon as an impression of a physical vibration is created in the mental realm, the body's innate intelligence is aware of it and responds to it, then this step has conceptual merit. In other words, while an impression doesn't "arrive at the mental realm" the way a mental impulse can certainly be said to "arrive at the tissue cell,"[89] the body's innate intelligence surely receives and responds to that impression. That

---

[87] Stephenson's *Chiropractic Textbook,* 1948 ed., Art. 92, p. 57
[88] *Ibid.* Art. 93, p. 58
[89] See *Step 12* above

it does, in fact, receive and respond to all impressions is evidenced by its perfect awareness of what happens to the body at all levels of vibration.

STEP 25: Mental (Realm)[90]

The twenty-fifth step of the Normal Complete Cycle is called *Mental,* which clearly refers to the Mental Realm, as described in Step 3, above.[91] This simply serves to remind us that we have now conceptually shifted planes of existence, and are considering the actions of intelligence again. Within the textual concepts of the Normal Complete Cycle, we actually entered the mental realm at *Step 22,* which we relabeled as *"Afferent Transformation."*

STEP 26: Interpretation[92]

The twenty-sixth step of the Normal Complete Cycle, called *Interpretation,* is also the sixth, and final, step in the more general Simple Cycle. This step denotes that the body's innate intelligence must perform an *operation* on any and all impressions (of the vibrations of the matter of the physical body) that it receives. In the analogy concerning impressions,[93] it was posited that an impression is like a footprint in the sand. The "foot" that leaves the impression is a vibration in the physical realm. The sand represents the *interface* between the physical and the mental realms, and more specifically the *receptivity* of the mental realm to changes in the physical realm. However, it was also noted that a depression in sand isn't actually a "footprint" until an intelligence, i.e. the observer, comes along, analyses it and recognizes it as such.

So it is with the body's innate intelligence and impressions. Impressions are the raw material of awareness. Each and every vibration in the physical realm creates a corresponding impression on the mental realm. This constitutes an unending stream of *potential* awareness. Actual awareness can only come from the intelligent operation of *interpretation.*

Interpretation is innate intelligence's analysis of what the impressions it senses denote. If you were looking at a footprint on a beach, you might say to yourself, "There is the big toe on one side. Those must be the smaller toes arranged in descending order to the left. That deep mark behind them was left by a heel striking the sand first. No claw marks like a bear's paw might leave – this is the left footprint of a human who passed by here." The awareness of the meaning of the impression is an outcome not just of the impression itself, but of the

---

[90] Stephenson's *Chiropractic Textbook,* 1948 ed., Art. 94, p. 58
[91] The addition of "Realm" to the title of Step 25, which is left out in Stephenson's *Chiropractic Textbook,* will make it consistent with the title of Step 3, and properly denote the connection between these two steps.
[92] Stephenson's *Chiropractic Textbook,* 1948 ed., Art. 95, p. 58
[93] See *Step 20* above

operation of my analytical intelligence.

So it must be with the body's innate intelligence, as it considers the impressions left by the vibrations of the physical body. One impression might mean that a hemoglobin molecule has just assimilated an oxygen atom. Another impression may indicate that a light photon just struck and changed the motion of a retinal rhodopsin molecule. A third that a biceps muscle cell just contracted, as it was instructed to do by a specific mental impulse from the body's innate intelligence. A fourth might indicate that a DNA nucleotide was just disrupted by a passing x-ray photon. This immaterial "interpretation" transforms each impression into a small bit of awareness concerning the state of the physical matter of the body.

> For example, one impression might mean that a hemoglobin molecule just assimilated an oxygen atom.

STEP 27: Sensation[94]

The twenty-seventh step of the Normal Complete Cycle is called *Sensation*. Stephenson's *Chiropractic Textbook* defines this as "what innate intelligence knows about one impression." As the physical realm undergoes a vibration (a unit of physical motion), the mental realm receives an impression of that vibration via afferent transformation, which the body's innate intelligence interprets to create a *sensation* (a unit of *immaterial awareness).*

The reduction of this process to individual "units" of consideration (i.e. one vibration producing one sensation) is purely a conceptual convenience on the philosopher's part. In order for us to model this living process intellectually, the Norman Complete Cycle describes the body's innate intelligence creating one specific mental impulse and sending it along a specific neural pathway to influence the adaptive response of a single specific tissue cell. Then, in the final efferent step (Coordination) Stephenson reminds the reader that, in actuality, the body's innate intelligence is creating countless mental impulses every moment, sending them along countless specific pathways to influence the adaptive responses of virtually all the cells of the innate body *simultaneously.*[95]

> The body's innate intelligence does not just perceive individual sensations from the body; it perceives an overall gestalt of the state of the body.

Similarly, the afferent side of the Normal Complete Cycle describes the nature of innate intelligence's awareness in artificially simplified terms. Changes in the body's state of organization are characterized by a single vibration creating a specific impression in the mental realm, which the body's innate intelligence interprets as a single sensation about the actions of the body expressing its own internal biological forces and/or the effects of an environmental force acting on

[94] Stephenson's *Chiropractic Textbook*, 1948 ed., Art. 96, p. 58
[95] See *Step 16* above

117

it. In reality, the nature of innate intelligence's awareness is just as *holistic* as the nature of innate intelligence's expression within the body. The body's innate intelligence does not just perceive individual sensations from the body; it perceives an overall *gestalt* of the state of the body, as well. To complete our "footprint" analogy, while you may muse analytically on the individually perceptible bits and parts of a footprint you are observing, the operational effect is that you see and respond to the footprint as a whole, complete thing, and even know something about the person who left that particular impression in the sand. So it is with the body's innate intelligence, which is aware of the whole body as a single, complete thing, and even knows something about the environment in which it is functioning!

STEP 28: Ideation

The twenty-eighth step of the Normal Complete Cycle is called *Ideation*.[96] "Ideation" is the name Stephenson gives to the mental picture that the body's innate intelligence creates from the summation of all the sensations it has of all the impressions it receives of all the vibrations of every material bit of the physical body.

Since the body's innate intelligence is *immaterial* and *limitless*, its *ideation* of the body can be complete, and its awareness perfect, from moment to moment. We can deduce the perfection of innate intelligence's ideation from three elements of our metaphysical speculation. First, the body's innate intelligence itself is assumed to be a perfect, infinite intelligence. Secondly, if any one vibration from the physical realm creates an impression in the mental realm, then *every* vibration must do so. And thirdly, impressions from the physical realm to the mental realm do not travel over physical pathways, and cannot be interfered with.

> For an organism to adapt, it must respond in such a manner as to return itself continually back to or toward wholeness.

Thus, if an infinite, perfect intelligence receives complete, perfect impressions of all the physical vibrations of the body, it will construct a perfect awareness of the actual physical state of that body.

The concept of ideation is crucial to an understanding of the reality of innate intelligence-driven adaptation. For an organism to adapt, it must respond in such a manner as to return itself continually back to or toward wholeness. To be able to do this, it must be aware of where and how its *actual form* deviates from its *ideal form,* which is that integrity of structure that allows it to maintain itself alive and functioning. Every adaptation is based first on an awareness of the actuality of the body's state of organization, then on the creation and expression

---

[96] Stephenson's *Chiropractic Textbook,* 1927,* Art. 97, p. 59
   *In the 1948 edition, the name of the step, "Ideation," was inadvertently left out of the title of Article 97. It is present in the original 1927 edition.

of an appropriate response, based on that awareness, to reorganize the body back toward an ideal, or at least a survivable, form. Ideation, a complete, perfect mental awareness of the body's actual state of organization, provides the basis for innate intelligence's response to the challenges facing the body.

STEP 29: Innate Intelligence[97]

The twenty-ninth step of the Normal Complete Cycle is called *Innate Intelligence*. We can easily dismiss the meaning of this step as just a reiteration of where we are conceptually and what the identity of the actor is. Since we have been closely following the progression from the physical realm (vibration) to the mental realm (impressions – interpretation – sensation – ideation), we are already perfectly aware that the body's innate intelligence is the "actor" at this point in the Normal Complete Cycle. This step serves only as a timely reminder of that fact.

On the other hand, we may wonder why Stephenson chooses to re-introduce the body's innate intelligence as the actor *at this point* in the cycle, when he has clearly been describing the actions of the body's innate intelligence since *Step 24*. A logical answer to this question is that this is the point where innate intelligence's role in function and adaptation changes from reactive to proactive, from afferent to efferent, from awareness to *response*. The step that follows this one, Intellectual Adaptation, is the actual bridge between awareness and response. It is simultaneously the *effect* of *Step 28* (Ideation – the complete awareness of the body that the body's innate intelligence obtains from its impressions) and the *cause* of *Step 4* (Creation – the creation of the specific adaptive messages (foruns) necessary to direct the next moment of adaptive response).

The reintroduction of the body's innate intelligence here also serves to illustrate that the adaptive response to follow does not originate from the body of a living organism. Rather the initial adaptive event is innate intelligence's *will to adapt*, which must then be impressed onto the matter of the physical body by the creation, transmission and expression of internal, biological forces, i.e. the efferent side of the Normal Complete Cycle. Thus, our perspective on the body's innate intelligence changes here from its ability to be aware to its *ability to respond*. Stephenson is introducing innate intelligence's **response-ability** (and therefore its primary *responsibility* for function, adaptation and health) right at this point.

STEP 30: Intellectual Adaptation[98]

The next step of the Normal Complete Cycle is called *Intellectual Adaptation*. As implied above, this step can be considered as the last step of the afferent side and/or the first step of the efferent side of the Normal Complete Cycle. It refers to

[97] Stephenson's *Chiropractic Textbook*, 1948, Art. 98, p. 60
[98] *Ibid.* Art. 99, p. 60

the action of the body's innate intelligence in light of its current ideation, which will be to form a plan for the response necessary to maintain the body and all its parts in optimum organization, or to return it back to its optimum organization.

This single step actually implies two distinct innate intellectual functions. The first is a comparison of the real (ideation, innate intelligence's awareness of the *actual state* of the physical body) to the ideal (the potential for total health, innate intelligence's awareness of how the organism ideally *needs to be organized*). The second is the comparison of the ideal (the *best possible* adaptive strategy) to the real (the adaptive response this organism *could actually make* at this moment in time). Both of these intellectual functions are implied in the concept of *intellectual adaptation,* although neither is named separately.

The first intellectual function is the final afferent function. In acquiring its ideation, its complete mental picture of the actual state of the organism, the body's innate intelligence has the ultimate afferent product, which we could conceive of as "whole body awareness." This awareness has no intrinsic value in and of itself. It can only have *adaptive value* if it can be compared to the fundamental adaptive value, namely the survival and expression of life in the current form of the organism. This necessarily implies a comparison between the actual state of the organism of the matter of the body and some yardstick of both minimal and optimal functionality.

The body's innate intelligence doesn't "know" standard physiological values. Rather it *sets the standard, moment by moment, for each individual.*

Thus we return to our understanding of the body's innate intelligence as the source of health, which literally refers to its role as the "author and creator" of the organizational template (DNA and enabling proteins) and pattern of life's unfolding (phenotype) in the first place. The body's innate intelligence holds the final authority of what is "normal." Thus, by comparing what is actual (ideation) to what is normal (ideal), it perceives what the variances are. The body's innate intelligence is also "that which establishes the difference" between what is and what should be. It doesn't "know" standard physiological values. Rather it *sets the standard, moment by moment for each individual.*[99] The simple way to put this is that in comparing its *ideation* to its *ideal,* the body's innate intelligence knows where the body's vibrational state is harmonious (at *ease)* and where it isn't (in *dis-ease).* Consequently, it knows in which direction it needs to influence each and every metabolic and functional vibration of each and every tissue cell in the body.

In this non-temporal instant, the body's innate intelligence does what it must do next. If we wish to attempt to conceive of this moment of intellectual adapta-

---

[99] Principle 26 – A living thing's innate intelligence is always normal, and its function is always normal, p. 79 above

tion, it is as if the body's innate intelligence performs a massive calculational algorithm for the variance from the optimum of every functional vibration and creates an exact compensatory correction for each variance proportional to that variance. Were the material body able to be nudged into making each and every compensatory correction its innate intelligence conceives, the net sum of these "corrections" would constitute an "ideal adaptive response." This, however, is not the entire story.

Secondly, the body's innate intelligence must compare this "ideal adaptive response" against its intimate, perfect and absolutely realistic awareness of the body's material resources, genetic potentials, and current state of structural and functional integrity. In other words, the body's innate intelligence must compare its perfect intellectual response against what it knows of the body's "limits of matter." If it had wings, a human being could fly from the roof of a burning building (and thus adapt successfully), but the body's innate intelligence must also know that this response, while perhaps ideal, is not possible. It must compare what the body *could do* to adapt against what it *can do* within its own material limits. Only then can it tailor the intellectual adaptation appropriate for the moment; i.e. the response to all the body's needs and challenges that the body can carry out *as it exists at that moment*. This becomes, as Stephenson puts it, the "plans of Innate to meet circumstances."[100] Of course, this plan exists only as an immaterial awareness of the direction the adaptive alterations of physiology must take. This *potential form* of an adaptive response is the same thing as the *information necessary to create such a response* within the physical matter of the body.

> The *potential form* of an adaptive response is the same thing as the information necessary to create such a response within the physical matter of the body.

STEP 31: Universal Intelligence[101]

Universal Intelligence, the *final step* of the Normal Complete Cycle, is also the *first step* of the Normal Complete Cycle. Its addition, here at the end of the cycle, merely indicates that the body's innate intelligence is the same "intelligence" as that universal intelligence responsible for organizing the entire universe. Thus, the cycle is complete and starts over again. Actually, the continuity of the Normal Complete Cycle goes directly from innate intelligence's *Intellectual Adaptation (Step 30)*, formed in response to its awareness of the current physical state of the body, to innate intelligence's *Creation (Step 4)* of the next cycle of mental impulses.

---

[100] Stephenson's *Chiropractic Textbook*, 1948 ed., Art. 99, p. 60
[101] *Ibid.* Art. 100, p. 63

CHAPTER 15

Conclusions

The conclusion of this process of review and deductive elaboration of the Normal Complete Cycle lies in the insight gained by the exercise itself. Clearly some elements of this analysis have required altering, renaming, rethinking or even deleting some steps of this model altogether. Nonetheless, we can conclude that the Normal Complete Cycle has much more to offer us in its logical validity, thoroughness and depth of consideration, than the exposure of some of the model's weaknesses could possibly undermine. The great and unappreciated strength of Stephenson's cyclic models (the Simple Cycle,[102] the Inter-Brain Cycle,[103] the Normal Complete Cycle, the Abnormal Complete Cycle[104]) is that they help us to consider how an immaterial, interactive, system-wide biological intelligence would have to operate to accomplish the ongoing, active and responsive adaptability that is so clearly manifested by living organisms. These models also place in our hands a practical metaphor for the crucial role *interference* plays to the detriment of normal function and therefore to the detriment of human health. This then becomes a compelling rationale for chiropractic's central focus on the phenomenology of the vertebral subluxation as a significant and perhaps pandemic source of subtle neurological interference, with its consequent incoordination *(dis-ease)* and lessening of the expression of the human potential for health, creativity, growth and evolution.

> **Chiropractic's approach to "health care," being based on these principles, will be radically different from any approach to health care that is based on a mechanistic metaphysical model of the universe.**

Finally, when we consider both the clearer, more organized metaphysical syllogisms described in the first part of this book, and the Normal Complete Cycle as we have just revisited it, we can't help but conclude that the chiropractic profession's approach to "health care," if based on these principles, will be *radically different* from any approach to health care that is based on a mechanistic model of the universe. A mechanistic doctrine tends to view the nature and therefore the

---

[102] *Ibid.* Art. 36, p. 7
[103] *Ibid.* Art. 112, p. 74
[104] *Ibid.* Art. 124, p. 83

very existence of the universe as a massive, strictly physiochemical process, driven by randomness and entropically tending toward maximum disorder, with life being nothing more than an improbable eddy of reverse entropy (enthalpy), coming about quite accidentally through the summative expression of the chemical properties of certain polymerized carbon compounds in the coincidental environment of the planet we happen to find ourselves occupying. When applied to the question of health and sickness, such mechanistic models tend to emphasize the character of living things as victims of, rather than adaptive to, the chaotic confluence of external forces acting on them. In chiropractic, this has long been characterized as the "outside-in" approach to health and sickness.

If we consider the microbes we live with and that live with us, this outside-in approach gives us the "germ theory of disease." When we look at the pollutants and stresses that bombard us from our environment, outside-in thinking produces a "stress-based theory of disease." The same philosophy, when applied to the "randomly accidental" quality of the genetic templates we all start life with (based on the random assortment of alleles during meiosis, and the random nature of the specific sperm/egg combination produced by fertilization mechanisms), produces the current shift toward a "genetic theory of disease." In all of these outside-in approaches, the living organism is seen as a victim of the germs (biological competitors) that infect it, or a victim of the physical and/or chemical forces (stressors) that continually bombard it, or even as a victim of the natural variations imbedded in its own genetic inheritance. As a consequence, all of these outside-in factors are conceived of as the focus of intervention, the "point of attack," in those health care approaches based on such mechanistic models.

Chiropractic's basic "intelligent substance" model *("intelligence, matter and the force which unites them"*[105]) considers questions of health and sickness from the perspective of both nature and life as fundamentally self-creating, self-maintaining, self-evolving and self-adapting. This informs a view of the living thing, not as just the product of the external forces acting on it, or of the "accident" of its own conception, but as an autonomous, self-aware and self-responsive (and therefore self-responsible) entity, creating and re-creating its own health moment by moment. We can refer to this view of life as a *vitalistic,* as opposed to a mechanistic, view. This makes "health" (the living thing's own self-created, continuously adaptive, coordinated functioning) the "natural state of being," and whatever interferes with the expression of this fundamental quality of life, the potential problem. Chiropractic has long characterized this as "inside-out" thinking.

As a consequence of this approach, clearly underlain and even more clearly supported by the very syllogisms revisited and revised above, chiropractic does

---

[105] Principle 6 – Any organized structure is a triunity having three necessary factors; namely, intelligence, matter and the force that unites them, p. 78 above

not offer another "theory of disease causation." Its philosophy leads inexorably to the conclusion that "innate intelligence-driven coordination/adaptation" is the true nature of health. Such a *vitalistic* philosophy also proposes that any *interference* with the transmission of the coordinative and adaptive internal, biological forces that would normally create and maintain the health of the organism, should be considered the primary cause of any incoordinated and maladaptive responses an organism might make to an impinging microbe, or to physical/chemical/emotional stresses, or even in the expression of the variations contained within its own genetic templates, that we characterize as sickness and disease. This approach can better be characterized as the "interference theory of mal-adaptation" than as a specific theory of disease causation, although chiropractic is neither first nor alone in positing mal-adaptation as a significant contributing factor in many "patho-physiological" states of being.

Thus, the *radically different* approach to health care that this syllogism suggests is to look to the individual's own natural vitality, his/her own adaptive potentials, in other words, the individual's own *innate intelligence,* as the primary healer, the source of each individual's own health, well-being, optimum functioning and healing. The challenge for any "health care provider," be it chiropractor or medical doctor, psychologist or shaman, is to recognize that the "health care provider" *cannot provide* the very health the "patient" seeks, because the locus of healing, health, and even life itself, lies within the "patient" and *not* with the "healer/doctor." This being truly accepted, the conclusion that the **best service** any "health care provider" can offer is to **help remove any interference or overcome any obstacles to the expression of this inexhaustible source of health and vitality,** rather than try to augment its efforts or supplant it outright, is inescapable. As we study the principles that form the basis for chiropractic's traditional metaphysical view of organization, life, health, awareness and response, a better understanding of their overall internal consistency and logical integrity can only help to *increase our confidence* in the actuality and potency of life's own perfect wisdom, its *innate intelligence.* It is this confidence that underlies the rationality of the inside-out approach to helping others achieve their own maximum expression of that internal wisdom, through the location, analysis and correction of the vertebral subluxation that we know as **chiropractic care.**

Chiropractic's basic "intelligent substance" model considers questions of health and sickness from the perspective of both nature and life as fundamentally self-creating, self-maintaining, self-evolving and self-adapting.

INDEX